# Tokyo Diet

How I lost 55Lbs on Japanese-American cooking

# Tokyo Diet

How I lost 55Lbs on Japanese-American cooking

## MIKIKO NAKAYAMA

TRANSLATED BY YASUYO BATTENFELD

To order additional copies of this book, contact:
Xlibris Corporation
1-888-795-4274
www.Xlibris.com
Orders@Xlibris.com
51542

# Contents

**Warnings about Eating American food and Guide to Eating Japanese food: Upshot from living in New York for 20 years**

I faced a crisis after the American size 2XL became too tight to wear because I had indulged myself eating American food. As I needed to solve this problem, I changed to eating Japanese food; and then, I lost 55 lb. I then realized how Japanese food was suitable for dieting. Had I changed to traditional Japanese food when the zipper on my jeans became much too tight and paid more attention for my health, I would not have become so overweight and could have been healthier.

Based upon the experience that I had switched to traditional Japanese food was the reason that I escaped from American style obesity, I wrote this book. I wish everyone who is overweight or overweight reservists to lose weight and become healthy. I weighed 175 lb. but lost 55 lb. (about 25 kg) and now weigh 120 lb. (about 54 kg). This is also a book warning myself that I will never become overweight again.

# In the Beginning

*Obesity grows in the United States*

*Reports from the Food Scene, and warnings about Consuming American food based upon my own experience*

As I have lived in New York City for a number of years, I found out one thing. When Japanese people eat American food more than three years, they tend to get heavier. As far as I know, Japanese, especially who have lived in New York, claim that they have gained weight. This is not an official statistic, but 28 out of 30 Japanese people claimed that they had gained weight.

While living in the United States, we naturally tend to eat American food and a lot of it! When you go to supermarkets in New York City and take a look at what they sell, it is self explanatory why we gain weight. Beef is much thicker than what we see in Japan. Whole chickens, not cut up pieces, are sold. Even if they are packaged, there are 5 or 6 large lumps. Some of the packages contain pieces which are equal to 2 or 3 whole chickens.

Compared to Japan, food prices are definitely cheaper. When you eat out, the amount of food served is so generous that Japanese people can barely finish all of them whether it is at a fast food or a regular restaurant. As you get used to it, however, they get used to the amount and eventually are able to clean up the plate. Although it has become relatively easy to get Japanese food nowadays, it is American food that can be purchased easily and cheaply. As we are not aware of it, American food takes a center place over Japanese food.

I have always loved Japanese food, especially a bowl of rice and miso (soy bean paste) soup, and I thought I would continue eating Japanese meals even after I began to live in the United States. Nevertheless, American food is cheaper than Japanese food, and it makes you feel full; furthermore, fast food is readily available and is inexpensive. Before I knew it, I was eating American food and I gained weight steadily. I am 168 cm, and I weighted 60 kg when I left Japan. I don't claim that I was a slim person, but I was not overweight. I thought of being fat had nothing to do with me. I was strangely certain that I would never be heavy after I arrive at the United States. Well, I gradually realized that I was no exception.

I stopped working as a freelance writer in Japan and came to the United States in 1987. I had planned to stay less than a year studying English as a Second Language, and I chose a private school, Wesleyan University, in West Virginia because there weren't many Japanese students in the area. I ate three meals at the school cafeteria. As the school fees included meals, I felt I had to eat; otherwise, I thought I would lose out. I could have chosen two meals instead of three meals a day, but I selected a plan with three meals. I was a foreign student, and I scarcely knew the area. The university offered a buffet breakfast. There were scrambled eggs, crispy bacon, sausages, ham, cornflakes, pancakes, French toast, waffles, droughts, hamburgers, toast, salad bar, various kinds of juice including orange juice, apple juice, cranberry juice, fruits in seasons, yogurt, coffee, tea, and such carbonated drinks as Pepsi and Coke.

Of course I didn't have to eat everything, but I was curious. Whatever I saw, I wanted to try. Since it was a buffet style, I ended up eating more than necessary. Apart from what were laid out, a chef holding a frying pan asked me what I wanted, and he cooked fried eggs, a cheese omelet and such. While not trying to speak English very much, I loved to eat. I was thrilled to have the food in the cafeteria. My American roommate did not make to the cafeteria as she was too sleepy to get up, but I went to the cafeteria and ate and ate. I actually thought it was wasteful not to eat breakfast since it was included in tuition. Different daily menus were presented morning and night including beef, chicken, fish, vegetables, pasta, bread and such. We were allowed to choose one dish from either meat or fish on the main menu. Ice cream, cookies, chocolate cake, cheesecake etc. were attractively laid out for lunch and dinner desserts. I was surprised of the enormous quantity of served food at first. They were about four times of the quantity of meals I ate in Japan. My breakfast had consisted of one scramble egg, sliced seaweed, miso soup and rice in Japan. In comparison, a minimum of two eggs for sunny-side up, and three eggs for scramble eggs or an omelet were used. I was pleased that I could eat eggs as much as I wanted. I felt that if I did not eat like Americans, I would not be as strong as they were; so, I ate and ate. English was difficult, and I understood little; and yet, I was not very tired physically. I was stressed out and needed food. I then realized that a mind needed nourishment even if a body was not very active. I gained 4 kg (8.8 lb) for a staying a year in the college.

The meals I could not finish eating at the cafeteria when I started living in the United States soon disappeared into my stomach very easily. Because they were buffet style meals, I could go back for seconds and thirds. I told myself, "I had to eat; otherwise, I would not survive this English hell." So, I continuously ate and ate. Only physical strength counts, and in order to gain physical strength, I thought I needed to eat. (I realize it is incorrect to say that physical strength is acquired simply by eating. However, I actually believed that notion back then.) Besides going to classes, I spent days eating at the cafeteria and studied at the library. Even though the college campus was big, my life consisted of moving among the cafeteria, dormitory and library. My jeans that I had worn in Japan didn't fit me anymore. Not only it was too tight, I could not pull it above my thighs. I gained 8 kg. (17.6 lb.). I left the dormitory and started to cook my own food, but the stomach which had been expanded couldn't shrink easily.

## Triggering Successful Diet

To lose weight is equally desired both in Japan and the United States, and a numerous advertisements for dieting are found in magazines, TV programs, and internet. Many new dieting methods appear one after another for a cycle of every 5 to 10 years. Atkins Diet was introduced by Robert C Atkins M.D. 10 years ago throughout the United States. It is indeed "a new diet revolution". A dieter can eat fat and meat as before, but he or she can rarely eat bread and pasta which are carbohydrates. This dieting method became a center of pros and cons throughout the United States. At the same time, Barry Sears PhD. proposed Zone diet. Dr. Sears, a leading scientist of biotechnology, insisted the necessity of avoiding taking carbohydrates. It maintained the insulin and the hormone balance because metabolism drained fat outside of a body by taking in fat. What has become popular recently is South Beach Diet, and it was suggested by Arthur Agatston M.D., Assistant Professor of Miami University. A dieter takes in good oil such as olive oil but avoids taking in bad oil, sugar and carbohydrates. However, chocolate is allowed for dessert, and it is a popular diet among Americans who like chocolate. Nevertheless, restricting of carbohydrates and such is required until the dieter hits the desirable weight, and rules are strict. For instance, even after the weight loss, one needs to eat non bleached bread. The Association of American Dieticians call them "fake diets" and general nutritionists do not recommend and support them.

I was desperate and attempted to lose weight. I was completely involved in dieting for the first week as I was very motivated. After one or two weeks passed, I started to suffer from sudden hunger pains and a strong desire to eat. My body could not cope with carbohydrate limitation. I could not stand hunger, and my hands started to shake. As if I was suffering from anemia, I felt giddy when I stood up. I felt very weak and I was about to faint; I could not stand it. I was on the rebound, and I ate and ate. After trying to diet a month or so, I failed trying all the diets. After I repeated these trials, I felt desperate. I was too fat and won't be able to go back to Japan as most of the Japanese people are not fat. I tried different kinds of diet and failed them each time. It is not likely that eating one type of food or a product makes you skinnier. I complained to myself that advertisements were fraud and one could not lose weight as easily as they claimed it to be.

When I failed a diet, I consoled myself and finally defended myself that there is nothing wrong with me being heavy as I am healthy. After having tried to be on a diet a number of times, I weighted a little less than 80 kg (175 lb.) My dress size was 2 XL, sizes 16-18, and my waist was over 1 meter. My panty, bra and shoe size were10, 44D, and 8.5W (wide width) respectively. We often use BMI (Body Mass Index) to measure, which is calculated by dividing weight by the square of height. I calculated as follows:

Weight 80 kg ÷ (1.68m x 1.68m) = 28.36. The reasonable BMI was below 18.5-25, which proved that I was definitely overweight. There were different levels of overweight: below 25-30 is the first degree, 30-35 is the second degree, 35-40 is the third degree, and over 40 is the forth degree, and under 18.5 is too skinny.

Besides MBI, we often speak about body fat percentage. It is measured by the percentage of fat over the body weight. In the past, we actually got into water and measured the body fat, but it is measured by electric resistance now. The body fat percentage of women is as follows: 20-25 are reasonable, 25-30 are slightly high, and over 30 is too high. Recently, a commercial scale with a tool that indicates body fat percentage is sold in stores. When I decided to go on a diet, I first bought this type of a scale. Even though I measured myself a number of times, it was always 31, which was pretty high. When one gains weight this much, it would become difficult to find a dress size in Japan.

## Incentive to lose weight

As everyone has a turning point, mine has also arrived. In 1990's, New York City was developing condominiums. It somewhat resembles to applying for a municipal apartment in Japan. I had applied for it, and I received a notice of acceptance 10 years later. I actually received the notice in July, 2005. My apartment was in Chelsea area in Manhattan. When I had applied, Chelsea was located at the edge of Manhattan. It was close to the warehouse area facing the Hudson River, and there was no shopping arcade nearby. It was a pretty rough area. After 15 years, however, progress has been made, and Chelsea has changed to a fashionable area next to Soho where art galleries and chic boutique shops are abundantly seen.

As I moved to Manhattan from the suburbs, I had to change my life style 180 degrees. At first, I needed to change my job in Manhattan. There are many differences living in Manhattan as opposed to living in the suburbs. At first, when you own a car, in addition to a monthly rent, you need to pay for a parking fee which is over $300 per month. If you do not rent a parking garage and park on the street, it is likely that you would get a parking ticket or a tow truck will tow away your car. The parking ticket is $150, and you have to be ready to pay for $300 for one time charge if your car is towed away. Having considered these issues, I came with a conclusion that it is not possible to own a car in Manhattan. After all, I am not rich at all. I moved into my apartment on August 15th, a month after receiving the letter of approval. About roughly 6 months later, the end of January, 2006, I was hired by a Japanese food company. On February 1st, I started my new job riding the subway in New York City after an interval of 12 years.

As I was used to driving a car, it was hard to walk everywhere. On the first day, I walked to the subway station for 5 minutes. I took the E train from the 23rd Street subway station and got off the train at the 52nd street on the 5th Avenue. I walked up 150 steps from the subway platform to the ground exit and panted heavily. I had not realized how heavy I was when I was driving a car; now that I took the subway and walked up and down the stairways, I realized my heaviness.

On the way to work, I was standing up and holding on to a strap. A woman sitting in the seat in front of me offered me a seat. "Won't you like to sit down? Is your baby about 7 months?" I was puzzled at first, but I then realized. It is apparent that the woman must have thought of me as pregnant as I was very fat. Although I accepted the seat, I felt blue. This was a turning point that I decided to lose weight. Dieting won't work simply if you want to look smarter and better. In my experience, you will work hardest when you have a strong desire and a specific objective.

# CHAPTER 1

# The basis of diet is what you eat

*For openers, check what you eat*

The fact that I was mistakenly taken as pregnant and was offered a seat on the subway and panted on the subway steps made me clearly realized that I was overweight. I decided to check what I have been eating. I wrote out what I have eaten in one day, and the following is an example.

Breakfast: 2 slices of toast, 2 Tbs of butter, 2 sunny-sides up eggs, 1 large banana, commercially prepared fruit yogurt 1 cup

Lunch: Store made sandwich called "hero sandwich" with liberal serving of ham, lettuce, sliced tomatoes and onions inside of skinny bread resembling French bread with mayonnaise on top together with a cup of clam chowder soup

Dinner: 2 large bowls of rice served liberally, one 8 lb. beef steak, vegetable salad with a generous amount of creamy dressing, a plate of potatoes cooked German style, a bowl of soup with liberal servings of sliced and cut pork and vegetables

Snack: a bag of potato chips, corn chips etc.

After roughly calculating my caloric intake, I was consuming 3,800 calories. Considering my weight, height and the amount I exercised, what I needed was 2,000 calories or so. If my intake is more than that, the rest is stored as fat in the body. I thought about ways to lose calories so that my caloric intake would be 2,000. I had thought about cutting down from 2 slices to 1 slice of toast and such, but I thought better of it to start from the beginning. Instead of cutting down what I ordinarily eat little by little, it seemed to make more sense to make a meal menu with 2,000 calories. It is up to a person how to distribute 2,000 calories, but I decided to do the following: breakfast 3 (600 calories), lunch 4 (800 calories), and dinner 3 (600 calories.) It is also advisable to do the following if you eat a snack or fruit: breakfast (500 calories), snacks twice a day for 100 calories each (200 calories), lunch (800 calories), and dinner 500 calories.)

**Use dietetics for dieting, but don't dwell on caloric calculation**
**Different body structure between Americans and Japanese**
**causes the difference of caloric intake**

The method of calculation in the U.S. uses ounces and pounds, so the Japanese method is not applicable. Those who need caloric calculation must obey the dietary regimen, and it gives a point of reference. Nevertheless, it is not a big issue. People with a strict dietary regimen must follow caloric intake, but it is inspected on a weekly basis, not on a daily basis in the United States. Even if a dieter goes a little overboard one day, but if he makes a weekly caloric target, it is considered acceptable in the United States. In Japan, on the other hand, dieters follow figures indicated by caloric calculation without fail. Caloric figures in Japanese hospitals are very exact. For instance, a Japanese hospital may set a standard at 1,840 calories, and a menu is planned accordingly. In the United States, a hospital will set a standard at 1,800 calories, but it won't be as detailed as 1,840 calories.

The calculation method to find out how much calorie a dieter needs differs between Japan and the United States. You may skip this section if numbers aren't your forte.

The Japanese-style equation for calorie intake may look like this.
Height (m) x height (m) x 22 = standard weight
Standard weight (kg) x intake energy for activity energy (KCAL) = intake energy for one day (KCAL)

For example, a person whose height is 165 cm is 1.65 x 1.65 x 22=59.895kg, which is roughly 60 kg. When a person's daily activities require modest energy, a seat work for instance, it is multiplied by 25 KCAL/kg. If the standard weight is 60 kg, it is calculated as 60 kg x 25 KCAL=1,500 KACL.

If a person's daily activities are moderate, it is multiplied by 30 KCAL/kg. If the standard weight is 60 kg, it is calculated as 60 kg x 30 KCAL=1,800 KAL.

If a person's daily activities are slightly higher such as doing some physical labor, it is multiplied by 35 KCAL/kg. If the standard weight is 60 kg, it is calculated as 60 kg x 35 KCAL=2,100 KAL.

There are a number of calculation methods in the United States, and the following is the most standard method. For men, weight x 24 hours are basic calories, and for women, weight x 0.9 x 24 hours are basic calories. Add exercise life active mass to these basic calories. In order to calculate exercise life active mass, multiply percentage to basic calories as follows: For low life active mass, multiply 20% by basic calorie, for slightly lower life active mass, multiply 55% by basic calorie, for moderate life active mass, multiply 70% by basic calorie, and for higher life active mass, multiply 80% by basic calorie. These numbers are added to basic calories, and the 10% of the total is added to the totaled calories.

For instance, for a 60 kg man, required daily calories are calculated as follows: 60 kg x 24 hours=1440 KCAL (basic calories). If his daily exercise life activity calories are moderate, multiply by 70%, 1440 KCAL x 0.7=1,008 KCAL (exercise life activity calories.) Add basic calories to exercise life activity calories, 1,440 + 1,008=2,448 KAL. 2,448 x 0.1=24.48 (10%) Add the 10% to the total, 2448 KCAL+24.48=2472.48 KCAL. So, approximate numbers of a total daily calories needed is 2,450 calories. Assuming the same weight, there are more calories in an American method than a Japanese method. As a matter of fact, I remember how surprised I was to find out that Americans take in many calories in 1998 which was a year I studied nutritional course. I felt that it was more than 1.5 time more than what I had heard of in Japan.

In January, 2006, a guideline for eating habits was revised, and reducing calorie intake by Americans by 10 to 20% was proposed; so, it has become closer to a Japanese standard. For 30-51 year old women, 2,200 KCAL was changed to 1,800 KCAL, and for men of the same age level, 3,000 KCAL was changed to 2,200 KCAL.

Americans have bigger frames than Japanese, and they are heavier. Because of that, their calorie intake is larger. However, recently, following the Japanese calorie index, the United States has shifted to show the lower calorie index. After all, even if you were

| Children | Calorie Range | |
|---|---|---|
| | Sedentary ⟶ | Active |
| 2–3 years | 1,000 ⟶ | 1,400 |
| Females | | |
| 4–8 years | 1,200 ⟶ | 1,800 |
| 9–13 | 1,600 ⟶ | 2,200 |
| 14–18 | 1,800 ⟶ | 2,400 |
| 19–30 | 2,000 ⟶ | 2,400 |
| 31–50 | 1,800 ⟶ | 2,200 |
| 51+ | 1,600 ⟶ | 2,200 |
| Males | | |
| 4–8 years | 1,400 ⟶ | 2,000 |
| 9–13 | 1,800 ⟶ | 2,600 |
| 14–18 | 2,200 ⟶ | 3,200 |
| 19–30 | 2,400 ⟶ | 3,000 |
| 31–50 | 2,200 ⟶ | 3,000 |
| 51+ | 2,000 ⟶ | 2,800 |

Japanese and live in the United States, it may be better for your health to calculate less calorie intake according to the Japanese way.

## Make use of an American food pyramid in making your own menu

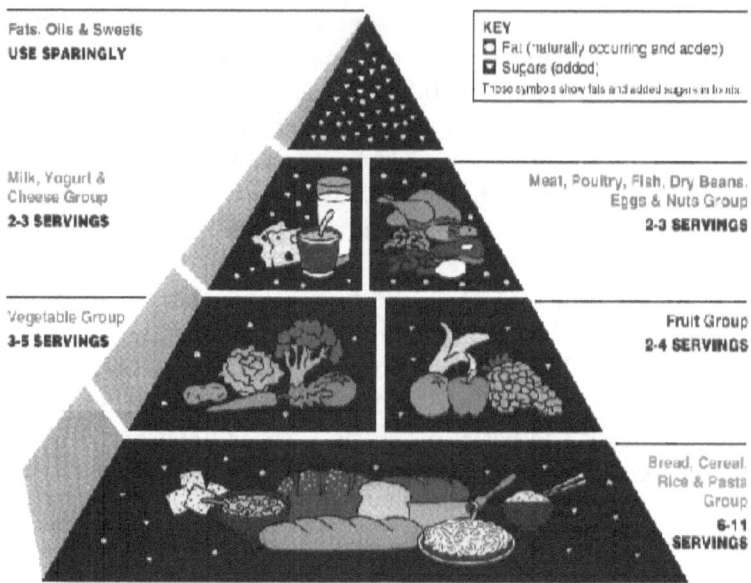

The food guide pyramid used for the nourishment instruction is classified into six areas: 1) fat and grease, and sugar, 2) dairy products made from milk, yogurt, and cheese, 3) meat and poultry, beans, eggs, nuts, 4) vegetables 5) fruit and 6) bread, cereal, rice, and pastas.

| Daily Amount of Food From Each Group | | | | | | | | | | | | |
|---|---|---|---|---|---|---|---|---|---|---|---|---|
| Calorie Level[1] | 1,000 | 1,200 | 1,400 | 1,600 | 1,800 | 2,000 | 2,200 | 2,400 | 2,600 | 2,800 | 3,000 | 3,200 |
| Fruits[2] | 1 cup | 1 cup | 1.5 cups | 1.5 cups | 1.5 cups | 2 cups | 2 cups | 2 cups | 2 cups | 2.5 cups | 2.5 cups | 2.5 cups |
| Vegetables[3] | 1 cup | 1.5 cups | 1.5 cups | 2 cups | 2.5 cups | 2.5 cups | 3 cups | 3 cups | 3.5 cups | 3.5 cups | 4 cups | 4 cups |
| Grains[4] | 3 oz-eq | 4 oz-eq | 5 oz-eq | 5 oz-eq | 6 oz-eq | 6 oz-eq | 7 oz-eq | 8 oz-eq | 9 oz-eq | 10 oz-eq | 10 oz-eq | 10 oz-eq |
| Meat and Beans[5] | 2 oz-eq | 3 oz-eq | 4 oz-eq | 5 oz-eq | 5 oz-eq | 5.5 oz-eq | 6 oz-eq | 6.5 oz-eq | 6.5 oz-eq | 7 oz-eq | 7 oz-eq | 7 oz-eq |
| Milk[6] | 2 cups | 2 cups | 2 cups | 3 cups | 3 cups | 3 cups | 3 cups | 3 cups | 3 cups | 3 cups | 3 cups | 3 cups |
| Oils[7] | 3 tsp | 4 tsp | 4 tsp | 5 tsp | 5 tsp | 6 tsp | 6 tsp | 7 tsp | 8 tsp | 8 tsp | 10 tsp | 11 tsp |
| Discretionary calorie allowance[8] | 165 | 171 | 171 | 132 | 195 | 267 | 290 | 362 | 410 | 426 | 512 | 648 |

It used to be a general instruction for a dieter to follow. It was a very general guideline indicating how many times each dieter should consume six areas of food per day indicated above, but this revision is more specific indicating how many cups or how many ounces a dieter should consume. For example, if a dieter is to consume 2,000 calories, he or she should eat 2 cups of fruit, 2.5 cups of vegetables, 6 ounces of grain, 5.5 ounces of meat and legumes, 3 cups of milk, and 6 teaspoonfuls of oil.

Base upon this, it is a good idea for a dieter, you, to make a one-day menu. The distribution of the food will become different depending upon how many times you are going to eat per day. You might eat four times a day including breakfast, lunch, snack, and dinner, or it might be five times a day if you eat snack before going to bed again. You need to divide calories based upon when and what you want to eat. In my case, I eat four times a day, and I eat a small portion for dinner and do not snack at night.

Example for 2,000 Kcal

| | Oil | Dairy product | Meat, poultry and fish | Vegetables | Fruit | Grain |
|---|---|---|---|---|---|---|
| Breakfast | 2 tsp | 1 cup | 1.5 oz | 1 cup | 1 cup | 2 oz |
| Lunch | 2 tsp | 1 cup | 2 oz | 0.5 cup | | 2 oz |
| Snack | | 1 cup | | | 1 cup | |
| Supper | 2 tsp | | 2 oz | 1 cup | | 2 oz |
| Total | 6 tsp | 3 cups | 5.5 oz | 2.5 cups | 2 cups | 6 oz |

Numbers are allotted in the chart, and you need to follow the amount of teaspoonfuls, cups and ounces where a total for each category is shown in the chart. For instance, a total amount of grain allotted per day is 6 ounces. When you divide this into breakfast, lunch, and dinner, it becomes 2 ounces per each meal. If grain is not eaten for lunch, you can eat 4 ounces of grain for supper. When your personal chart is completed, you then think about a menu you like to have.

When there is not enough time to eat rice and Miso soup for breakfast, you can eat 2 slices of toast (1 ounce per a slice) with 2 teaspoons fu of butter, a cup of milk, 1 egg and a slice of ham, one cup of broccoli, one small banana. If there is no time for toasting bread, have a cup of cereal (2 ounces) with milk and slice a banana as topping. You can drink a glass of 100% vegetable juice. Meat and fish may be consumed at lunch or dinner. Flexibility is needed; there is no problem when all the food you are supposed to eat is eaten in a day.

Food Exchange Lists are well known in Japan. Similarly, diabetics in the United States can exchange types of food within the same food group. (See the following chart)

You can make your own menu by selecting cereal, donuts, or crackers rather than choosing bread within the same food group.

**Food Exchange Lists**

**Carbohydrate (starch)**

| | |
|---|---|
| Cereal | 1/2 cups |
| Rice | 1/3 cups |
| Pasta | 1/2 cups |
| Corn | 1/2 cups |
| Mashed potatoes | 1/2 cups |
| Bagel | 1/2 cups (1 oz.) |
| A slice of bread | 2 slices |
| Muffin | 1/2 |
| Roll | 1 (1 oz.) |
| Rye bread | 1 slice |
| French bread | 1 slice |

**Meat**

| | |
|---|---|
| Beef | 1 oz. |
| Pork | 1 oz. |
| Chicken | 1 oz. |
| Fish | 1 oz. |
| Shellfish | 2 oz. |
| A can of tuna | 1/4 cups |
| Oyster | 6 |
| Cheese (cottage cheese) | 1/4 cups |
| Cheese | 1 oz. |
| Egg | 1 |

**Fruit**

| | |
|---|---|
| Apple | 1 |
| Banana | ½ |
| Blackberry | 3/4 cups |
| Melon | 1 cups |
| Grapefruit | ½ |

| | |
|---|---|
| Orange | 1 |
| Mango | ½ |
| Kiwi | 1 |
| Watermelon | 1 + ¼ cups |
| Peach | 1 |
| Strawberry | 1 + ¼ cups |
| Orange juice | ½ cups |

**Milk**

| | |
|---|---|
| (skim/Whole) | 1 cup |
| Yogurt | 8 ozs. |

**Fat**

| | |
|---|---|
| Butter | 1 tsp |
| Margarine | 1 tsp |
| Bacon | 1 slice |
| Sour cream | 2 tbsp |
| Vegetable oil | 1 tsp |
| Mayonnaise | 1 tsp |
| Salad dressing | 1 tbsp |

The problem is the amount you are going to eat. A slice of bread has 1 ounce, which is 28.3g. (**A loaf of Japanese bread which is sliced into 6 slices has 100 grams for each slice. The size of bread sold at the U.S. supermarkets is one quarter of Japanese bread, and it is rather light bread.**) Both one half of a bagel and a slice of pancake, 4 inches in diameter, contain 2 ounces, and a small muffin contains 1.5 ounces. It would be ideal if you weigh each item; but if not, you can switch a bowl of rice to two slices of bread. If you are aware of items you can exchange, you should not become too nervous. Basically, it is the same for meat which belongs to a protein group. An approximate size of chicken, beef, mackerel and tuna etc. that are equal to the size of a palm of a hand is 3 ounces. Although fatty beef and fatless breast of chicken have different nutritional value, you might like to remember as a good size is what can be placed on a palm of a hand. If you become too nervous and are concerned about weight too much, your meal will not be tasty. You need to take portions described in each group and make your own well balanced menu while enjoying doing so. I repeat that what you must do is that you should consult from each group from the food pyramid. You then distribute them into 4 meals per day, think of your favorite menu, and enjoy eating them.

## The standard meal plan in the United States

Breakfast: 1 cup of milk (low fat), 1 cup of orange juice, ½ cup of cereal, 1 slices of non breached bread toasted with 1 tsp margarine

Lunch: One tuna fish or turkey sandwich with 2 ounces of meat with 2 tsp of mayonnaise, tomato, and ½ cup of lettuce, made with 2 slices of non breached bread. One apple, a cup of milk or one yogurt, and coffee

Dinner: 3 ounces of T-bone steak which may be substituted with chicken or fish, ½ potato, 1 cup of broccoli, 1 cup of kiwi which may be substituted with strawberries, melons etc. and coffee

Snack: 3 crackers with 1 tsp of cream cheese

This is only a guideline. There is no need to force yourself to eat something you do not care to or do not like to eat. It becomes nutrients as you enjoy eating them. Needless to say, it is most important to have a good balance; however, even if you do not eat what you do not care for, there is always something you can substitute with. For instance, if milk is not your favorite, substitute with cheese, soybean milk or yogurt. Combining these foods well and you will make your own favorite menu.

## Esthetic appearance rather than counting calories

At first, I was very much into counting calories. I placed everything on the scale whether it may be fish, vegetables, or rice and solemnly counted calories. While cooking, I placed a measurement cup and spoon in front of the counter. I then cooked following instructions. When a day ended, I wrote a journal and made a menu for the next day. I counted calories and followed exactly the way it should be. Because many computer software programs are available nowadays, it is not necessary to count calories using a calculator. You simply have to type in the menu and amounts, calorie counts will be displayed. Actually, when you count all the ingredients of the menu you eat, you can pretty much figure out the rough numbers just by looking. I then decided that I do not need a scale any longer on my own. It would be better if you can continue counting calories, but I am too lazy and sloppy. So, I decided to trust my gut feeling.

Actually, as you go on with your daily life, it is not realistic to weigh fish, meat each time you eat. Many people might feel that it is too troublesome to count calories. While eating out, we cannot find out what type of ingredients each restaurant is using as well as its cooking method. Then, it is not possible to count calories in a strict sense. I therefore gave up counting troublesome calories, and I decided to focus on the amount of food intake.

## Eat 60 g of carbohydrates per serving, and eat a small amount of supper

To start out, you need to lower the amount of rice you eat. There are many kinds of diets such as breakfast less or supper less diet. As I have a big appetite and cannot start a day without breakfast, it was hard not to eat breakfast. On the other hand, I did not want to cut down the amount of lunch as it sustained my activity level for midday. So, I decide to eat less supper. I had loved eating full meals and had thrived on food, especially rice, but I cut down the amount of rice intake. I reduced from eating two bowls of rice to one bowl; furthermore, the amount of rice in the bowl was cut down in half. I also cut down the size of rice bowl from a large china bowl size to a small size generally used by women while I did not pack rice but served myself lightly. A dinner plate was also reduced from a large plate with a diameter 27.8 inches to a medium plate with a diameter less than 20 inches, and I tried not to give myself a liberal helping of food on it. I always had soup or miso soup while I increased a number of plates. There I served myself vegetables boiled and seasoned with sugar and soy sauce, salad, vinegared kelp and mushrooms, etc. I avoided a bowl of rice with a topping including a pork cutlet or curried rice, which inevitably decreased the amount of carbohydrates intake. The amount of pasta, noodles, rice and my favorite, potatoes, was decreased to half of what I used to eat. Even though I was eating more than two big china bowlfuls of rice which weighted more than 400g, I cut down to 200g. I stopped taking snack which had been consumed after dinner, sweets enjoyed at 10 in the morning and 3 in the afternoon, especially cake or ice cream until I start to see some effects.

## Sugar is taboo, and says No to sweets

I tried not to eat sweets as much as I could during dieting. If anything, I am a sweet tooth, and I always kept cheese cake, Japanese buns with sweet bean pastes in them, sweet bean jelly and such on the table as snack. As Japanese sweets were difficult to find, I actually made them. I justified myself that sweets were good for me to resolve my stress, and I snacked these sweets twice a day, or sometimes three times a day.

As sugar, especially white sugar, is refined, nutritious value is minimal, and it is one of the causes for obesity. I tried not to use sugar for my cooking, and I made sure to check the product labels and learned about the amount of sugar in the products. Diet instructions in the United States recommend that dieters must check the amount of carbohydrates rather than the amount of sugar. Sugar is contained in drinks and snacks, but our bodies do not consume a huge amount of sugar. However, we consume too many carbohydrates from rice, pasta and such without realizing it and the intake of carbohydrates are changed into monosaccharide and tend to be restored within the body. The methods of diet recommended in the United States are based on this reason that losing carbohydrates would reduce weight even temporarily.

Even though carbohydrates eventually change to monosaccharide, they take time to be resolved, and it is absorbed slowly. Because sugar is easily absorbed, it is better for a dieter to select items with less sugar when dieting.

Since I had decided to go on a diet, I made objectives. After all, I am not going to diet all my life and I only had to bear with it until I lose weight. It would be a matter of a few months. My first objective was aimed for the first three months. After that, I am going to make another objective. As I started my diet in March, I assumed that I would solve my three folded stomach; and then, I would be wearing a swim suit in the summer.

Nevertheless, I still wanted some sweets on snack time. Since eating snacks was a habit, I had to eat something. So I chose a snack made of agar-agar instead of sweets. Since it is kelp, it contains neither carbohydrates nor fat. As there is no calorie in it, it is effective as diet food. The food made of agar became the fad in Japan, and powdered agar (like gelatin), which is very convenient, became available. So, I decided to make a large amount at one time and eat them little by little. A cupful of agar is one portion. Cutting them into cubes, I scatter dried kelp and eat them with juice pressed from bitter oranges. The flavor is different from sweet dessert, but I told myself that I had to bear with it for only three months. The funny thing is that agar tasted well after all.

I also cut vegetables such as celery, carrots, and cucumbers into sticks, put them in a plastic bag, and carried wherever I went. I ate them instead of sweet snacks. The vegetables contain a lot of vitamins and a few calories; because of that, they are necessity for dieters. Dried nuts are also convenient to carry around, but there are too many calories if you overeat them. These snacks helped me when I was hungry and felt like eating "real" snacks.

## Read labels

I am a nutrition consultant, and perhaps because of my occupation, I always read food labels. Actually, I enjoy reading labels. For instance, yogurt contains different amount of sugar depending on manufacturers. DANNON Light and Fit, my favorite, has the following contents: weight 170 g (6 oz), fat 0g, no added sugar, 60 kg calorie. The label has 7 g. In case of AXELROD, the following contents are shown: weight 170 g (6 oz), fat 0 g, sugar 11 g, 90kg calorie. They are relatively low in sugar. When the labels indicate "organic" or "bean curd yogurt", they seem healthier. But when you carefully read the labels, there are many products that contain over 24 g of sugar. It is a common sense to read labels carefully and buy products in the United States.

There is so much sugar difference even in a single item, yogurt, so I decided to read labels of other commodities. Even for carbonated water, some of them contain sugar. A package indicates "sugar free", but if you read a label carefully, it is rare to find 0 g of sugar. In many cases, it contains a little bit of sugar. I was buying products simply by looking at prices, but my ways have changed after I went on a diet. The contents of fat, sugar, carbohydrates became more important than prices. The key words for dieting are fat free, no sugar added and low carbohydrates.

## Suppressing hunger pain by drinking morning homemade vegetable juice

I had been eating a tremendous amount; and yet, I drastically reduced the amount I took in. Of course, I suffered from hunger pain. Hunger wakes me up in the morning. I had devoured breakfast until I began dieting. But, I cannot expect the result of dieting had I eaten a huge breakfast then. So, I decided to suppress my hunger pain by drinking homemade vegetable juice. Just a word of caution is that I did not drink readymade juice. They contain too much sugar and are not fit for dieting. So, I decided to make my own stamina diet juice. I put a banana, a cup of soy milk, a teaspoonful of vinegar, and green vegetables such as celery and spinach into a blender and mix just for a few seconds. If green vegetables are not at hand, substitute instant green tea powder or green vegetable juice power. For those who cannot drink unless it is sweetened, you can add a teaspoonful of honey into it.

After I get up, I drink a glass of juice, and my hunger pain subsides. As a matter of fact, it also has many benefits. Potassium contained in bananas regulates the water balance of a body and keeps normal heartbeat. It also helps to relieve lethargy and weariness caused by muscle weakness. While lecithin found in soybeans is well known to lower cholesterol, soybeans contain abundant estrogen (female hormones). So, it is said to be effective to ease menopausal unpleasantness. Saponin which decreases lipid peroxide is found in soymilk in an easily absorbable form into a body, and it promotes blood run smoothly which prevents aging such as arteriosclerosis,

Vinegar lubricates citric acid cycles. Because green vegetables contain the vitamin B and C families which help smooth the metabolism of bodies, they help to solve the lack of stamina and irritability.

So, this juice is the basis for health. Dieting does not necessarily mean that you only lower calories.

## American meals are high in fat content

Essentially, it is ideal to have Japanese style breakfast. It is the best balanced meal to eat kelp and Japanese daikon (radish) miso soup, rice, greens seasoned with soy sauce, laver and small fish for breakfast, but there is no time to prepare this when you are busy working. In comparison, American style breakfast is easy to prepare. It is most convenient to have toast, a bagel, a muffin, droughts, or cereal with milk and coffee. As there are many New Yorkers who are of Jewish descent, we tend to see people who always eat a bagel. There many kinds of bagels: plane, cinnamon, raisins, sesame, blueberries, cherries. You dab cream cheese or butter. I used to love eating cinnamon and /or raisin bagels topped with a plenty of cream cheese. However, animal fat is high in cream cheese, so cholesterol is high as well. It is better to switch to vegetable fat for dieting. So I changed from cream cheese to peanut butter. I was persistent to check the sugar content when I bought peanut butter sold on the market. Even though it was labeled as fat free peanut butter, the sugar content varies. Since "sugar 0 g" is not available, I buy those with 3 to 7 g. Depending upon supermarkets or organic specialty shops, you can put peanuts or other nuts into a machine and make your own nuts and peanuts butter. As there are no additives in them, it is absolute natural food; it is gentle to your body.

The weight of bagels sold on the market varies depending on their brands. Bagels sold on supermarkets are usually priced two for $1.00 or 60 cents per one are shaped fairly big, but they are inflated, and they lack moist but chewy qualities, unique to bagels. A $2.99 five bagels in a bag made and sold by a large bread manufacturer may be handy, but it is not very tasty due to additives. Nutrition facts are shown on a bag or box of manufactured products, and it makes easier for dieters to calculate calories. As I had decided to eat a less amount, I wanted to choose a tastier one. What I recommend are bagels from bagel specialty shops. When you buy a bagel fresh from the oven, it is so delicious that it makes everyone love bagels. While living in Japan, I absolutely loved rice; I rarely wanted to eat bread. Nevertheless, as I ate bread fresh from the oven sold in any bakeries in New York, I came to realize that bread was not too bad. Needless to say, there are bakeries you can buy bread fresh from the oven in Japan as well, they were so soft including toasting bread that I did not like it. There are many kinds of bread in bakeries in New York. There are many kinds of flour: wheat, rye, whole grain wheat and millet. Blueberries, cranberries, walnuts, cashew nuts, sesame seeds, and so on are mixed in with dough. There are also different types of bread: French bread, rolled bread, toasting bread etc. These facts convinced me that staple diet in the United States is bread.

I used to eat a whole bagel of which weight is about 200 g, but now I cut a bagel in half of which weight is about 100 g. Spreading one teaspoonful of peanuts butter on the bagel, I consume about 80 kg calories. Since I drink my morning special juice, I barely feel hungry. I then eat yogurt. A word of caution is that calories of the manufactured yogurt differ from 70 kilo calories to 160 kilo calories.

## Meal time and chew 30 times

It is easier to diet if a dieter eats meals at the same time because a body is ready to take in meals. In other words, digestive and breathing functions are well prepared for the action. If a meal time becomes irregular or eats late at night, a dieter gets too hungry and tends to have a big meal, which causes overeating and bodily functions are less active. The fundamental of diet is to eat regularly and slowly. Incidentally, I was eating three times as much and as fast when I was heavy. Thinking back on it, I practically washed down and rarely chewed. As I was very busy, I washed down one dish meal with rice. For instance, there were boiled rice with an organic raw egg or hot green tea poured over cooked rice. I also ate a bowl of rice with a pork cutlet (with an egg), tempura or curry on top.

As I reduced the amount of food, it would disappear quickly if I did not chew thoroughly. So, I chewed a minimum of 15 times. I also decided to allow myself to take a longer meal time. My old-fashioned father used to say that eating fast is a skill one can learn, and he trained me to eat as quickly as I can. Because of that, I had a habit of eating in 5 minutes, but I changed my lifestyle to allow myself to have meals at least 30 minutes. I slowly drank my special vegetable juice and chewed a half bagel, salad and yogurt for the busy mornings. I chewed thoroughly at any rate.

In the beginning, I felt irritated, but I became so used to it that I no longer feel satisfied unless I chew thoroughly. The more you chew, the fewer amounts you need to eat for feeling full. As I chewed more than 15 times, my taste buds began tasting the natural flavor of food. It was the same thing even for salad. I have begun to taste the natural sweet flavor of vegetables. Because of it, I began choosing very fresh vegetables so that I can taste more sweetness of vegetables.

## Control yourself through your dinner

Everyone's metabolism is different, so I cannot make generalizations, but reducing the amount of dinner I consume became very effective in my case. According to American dietetics, one can maintain health for smooth digestion and absorption by eating three balanced meals. A menu is quite often made based upon the following rate: one (300-400K cal) for breakfast and two (600-800 Kcal) for lunch and supper. The principle of dieting is to reduce the amount of excess food which had been eaten and take out as the excess fat from a body. In my case, I was consuming only 300 Kcal in the morning, and it was difficult to reduce more calories from that. As there are those who cannot eat breakfast at all, I thought that a meal plan must be made according to one's constitution and lifestyle, and you had to play it by ear.

I had thought about it, and I decided to run a review of my dinner. If I become too hungry after dinner, I could go to bed. Of course, if you are too hungry, you might not get to sleep . . . . I realize it is not quite correct based upon dietetics, but I decided to lose carbohydrates eaten at dinner as much as I can. Although I was eating 2 to 3 big bowls of rice for dinner, I decided to use a smaller rice bowl made for children; I served myself one bowl of rice very lightly.

My stomach had been enlarged because of overeating, so it could not have satisfied with a smaller amount of a meal. Instead of rice, I decided to satisfy myself with less caloric vegetables and soup. After you drink a large bowl of soup at first, you tend not to eat much. You chow more than 15 times as I have noted, and you tend to feel fullness. As my brain might have directed the feeling of fullness while chewing, I gradually felt full. In 2 to 3 weeks, I felt very full after I had soup served in a regular cup or soup plate.

## Eat your supper early and stop eating after 8:00 p.m.

It does not seem to make any difference what time you eat as we are consuming the same nutrition, but the time you eat make a big difference for the sake of obesity. Especially, eating a late dinner causes a problem. Essentially, it is a time for a body to rest, but your stomach is absorbing what has been consumed. As the sugar in blood is not fully utilized as energy, it transforms to fat, and this fact accumulates. On the other hand, if you eat meals at a regular time, your body system digests and absorbs accurately and prepares it to become energy. As often said, the reason not to eat after 8:00 at night is that the food consumed then will be stored within a body. If you need to eat after 8:00 at night, it should be water based food such as soup, and you should not overeat. When you eat later than usual, you become very hungry, and you tend to overeat. Likewise, eating the amount of snack might increase, and it will increase calories as well. A lot of carbohydrates and sugar are found in snacks; if you need to have snacks, it is recommended to have low caloric items such as vegetables, agar products, etc.

## Animal fat is a taboo

A dieter should avoid animal fat to the utmost as it contains extremely high calories. After coming to the United States, I ate more meat as it was much cheaper compared to Japan. I ate fatty beef or pork at least once a week. I had thought that animal fat was the basis for energy. I used pork loin, not pork fillet to make port cutlet, and I enjoyed its fatty flavor.

Whether you are dieting or not, it is highly recommended for middle aged people not to eat beef or pork fat which are full of unsaturated fatty acid and cholesterol. I could not have ever imagined in the past, but I switched to buy chicken or turkey of which has less fatty parts. I decided to wait to buy beef or pork until the effect of dieting starts to appear. I removed chicken fat excluding breast meat prior to cooking. I checked the amount of fat and cut out visible fat, so it took me longer to cook.

## Focal point of dieting (Be careful with manufactured fried food.)

Regarding the oil used for my cooking, I carefully selected kinds of oil and checked labels. There is not 100% perfect oil; nevertheless, saturated fatty acid which solidifies in room temperature is mostly found in animal fatty acid, and unsaturated fatty acid which is liquid at room temperature is mostly found in vegetable oil. There are two kinds of unsaturated fat: monounsaturated fat and polyunsaturated fat. They tend to lower LDL (low-density lipoprotein) which is bad cholesterol as it adheres to blood vessels, and they tend to increase HDL (high-density lipoprotein) which is good cholesterol as it makes the flow of blood smooth.

The FDA recommends that the total fat intake should be limited to the 30% of all the food a person takes in, and it would be better to take monounsaturated fat. The following items contain monounsaturated fat: olive oil, macadamia nuts, canola oil, peanut butter and such. Even though they are vegetable oil represented by linoleic acid and such, the following items contain more than 50% of polyunsaturated fat in its entirety: safflower oil, sunflower oil, corn oil, soybean oil and such. Even though polyunsaturated fat lowers bad cholesterol in blood, it accelerates oxidation in a body and promotes to produce free radicals which damage cells. So, if would be problematic to take polyunsaturated fat too much. A word of caution here is that even FDA approved monounsaturated fat is not perfect. For instance, 77% of olive oil contains monounsaturated fat, but 14% contains polyunsaturated fat. All vegetable oil does not mean that it is all fine. When dieting, one should not consume too much oil, so I was very careful not to consume much oil. I decided not to eat tempura, pork cutlet and fried food even though they were cooked with vegetable oil during dieting.

## Controlling the amount to eat and what you eat when eating out

So, you are on a diet, and you stay home and eat your own diet meals. Well, this will interfere with your wellbeing, and the purpose of diet is to lose weight pleasantly. It does not last long without if you are too concentrated on dieting. The secret of dieting is working in cooperation with people around you. So, it is necessary to eat out sometimes with your friends. But, you cannot eat anything you want; the realization of a fact that you are on a diet is important. Special care makes a big difference for your calorie intake.

First, you should omit fried food, and you choose meat with less fat, i.e. fillet or chicken breast. You would rather choose fish than meat. Many restaurants are fully equipped with vegetarian menus. When eating out, it is best to select dishes with vegetables including salad and steamed vegetables. Regarding salad dressing, you could choose vinegar and olive oil and adjust it to your liking. Certain restaurants specify total calories and fat content, especially the amount of Trans fat. If not specified, you might like to ask about it. When ordering your meal, you could ask not to add cheese on salad or you might ask salad dressing separately as well.

# CHAPTER 2

# Dieting with American Style Japanese food, Ame-Japa meals

### Basics is Japanese meals

When I was in Japan, I had never thought that Japanese food was nutritionally best. I was dreaming to include Western meals, especially Italian, French and such in my diet. I was amazed and thrilled to find out the enormity of breakfast at the restaurant in Los Angeles Airport where I first landed in the United States. A large heavy meal signified a big country, the United States, and I honestly believed that it was the meal I had waited for a long time. Other Japanese students complained about the enormity of size, but I boasted that I could eat it all. I told them, "If you cannot eat it, we will be defeated by Americans." Other Japanese students regarded me with suspicion. The bigger the better was the motto of the fast food scenes in the 1980s in the United States. Hamburgers were twice as big as those in Japan, and the cups for coffee and carbonated drinks such as Coke or Pepsi were huge. At first, I was curious, and American hamburgers without any vegetables in it felt rich in comparison to Japanese hamburgers of which meat was combined with onions and bread crumbs. I had thought eating meat equaled to rich meals, but I was retaliated with becoming heavy, and once again, I saw a Japanese meal in a new light. The very basic of nutrition, balanced meals, was found in Japanese meals.

A hamburger has beef, bread, cheese which are animal fat, animal protein and carbohydrate, but it lacked vegetables. A hamburger comes with French fries, but it is more carbohydrate than a vegetable. Besides, it is fried, and it contains quite a bit of fat. In comparison to American meals, Japanese meals

---

31

have much less amount of fat. For example, an ordinary breakfast includes rice, miso soup, natto (fermented soybeans), dried laver, and pickled vegetables. The ingredient includes soy beans, seaweed, vegetable protein such as miso and natto, carbohydrate, and vegetables. They scarcely contain animal fat, and yet it has a good nutritional balance. You might say that it may be related to a meal menu.

When you see the way Japanese eat their meals, most Japanese people eat rice, side dish, miso soup alternately. In other words, they eat meals with a good balance. On the other hand, Americans concentrate on and finish with one dish first before moving on to another one. If they start with salad, they finish it first and move on to a hamburger. I do not mean to deny an American way of eating completely. As Japanese or American Japanese people cannot have the same eating habits as they are in Japan, it is best to prepare American style Japanese food. They should utilize American ingredient and cook Japanese style food which is suitable to American climate that is Ame-Japa meals.

## Japanese meal is balance food

An American acquaintance told me that Japanese food is healthy. Japanese food was introduced as well balanced meals in Nutrition class in the State University of New York. There are many Americans who strongly believe that Japanese food is good for health. I myself did not realize how true this is until I began living in the United States. Because I had immersed myself in American food, I gained some valuable experience.

It is an indelicate thing to mention, but I now compare what happens to your bowl movement after you switch to Ame-Japa meals. When I was eating American food, I had to strain myself to relieve myself. After switching to Ame-Japa meals, my excrement did not look like those of rabbits, and I did not have to strain myself. Because of that, my bleeding hemorrhoid has stopped, and I felt good. As you eat breakfast, I felt energetic. I had a full realization of being Japanese. It is important to lose weight, but it is meaningless if you get sick because of a diet. I decided to include Japanese food into my diet.

The superior quality of Japanese food has been written up in a number of books and newspapers, and it is probably not necessary to mention it here. Nevertheless, because of the longest life expectancy in the world, research on Japanese food has been carried out. Reflecting the results of research, Americans are showing a great interest in Japanese food. A basic food menu for Japanese food consists of eating rice, soy beans, fish and seaweed, and that seems to be the key to health.

## The Key to Health: Traditional Japanese meal in Okinawa Prefecture

According to Japanese Government, there are 457 people in Okinawa prefecture who are over 100 years old, and this is the world record. There are 34.7 people over 100 years old per 100,000 people as opposed to 10 people per 100,000 people in the United States. This comparison shows us there are many people who live a long life. The average lifespan in Okinawa is 81.2 years old; 86 for women and 78 for men. There are 6 people who are over 100 years old among the entire population of 3500 people in Ogumi village, which is known as a longevity village. Okinawan elders are not just living a long life, but also they are enjoying active life. *The Okinawa Program* researched the life style of Okinawan elders for 25 years, and it was on the best seller list in the United States. One of the authors, Craig Willcox Ph.D gave hope to many Americans. According to him, the amazing Okinawa report is based upon Okinawans eating good food; they eat a lot of potatoes and pork. It is closer to American meals than traditional Japanese meals. Americans can follow this eating habit, and the food is available in the U.S.A. In other words, if Japanese living in the U.S.A. eats Okinawa style American food, there is a possibility for them to become healthy and live a long life. Furthermore, the author mentioned that by eating Okinawan food, it would significantly lower the rate of people becoming cancerous as follows: 80% of vascular heart disease, 86% of prostate cancer, 82% of breast cancer, 57% of ovarian cancer and other cancers. He also added that many nursing homes would be out of business if this is realized.

In comparison with American meals, *The Okinawa Program* views that the traditional Okinawan meals contain more grain, fish, and vegetables, and less meat, eggs, and dairy products. However, Japanese people view this a little differently. Professor Ryoichi Taira of Ryukyu University has researched epidemiology of Ogumi village more than 15 years, and he analyzes the reasons of longevity as follows:

1) Salt intake by villagers is small.
2) The ratio of vegetable and animal protein intake is 1 to 1. Vegetable protein is consumed mainly from soy bean products and bean curd, and animal protein is mainly consumed from pork. The balance between eating meat and fish is good.
3) The salt intake in Okinawa is 9 g per day, which is the least number in Japan. The people in Tohoku area are known for their high salt intake, and the difference is clear that their salt intake is 14-15 g per day. The maximum salt intake suggested by Ministry of Health, Labor and Welfare is 10 g, and Ogumi villagers consume less than this amount.

4) Elders of Ogumi village consume an average 50 g of pork per day, and every part of pork from head to toe is utilized. It is cooked very slowly, and fat is scooped up. This cooking method is healthy, and cooking every part of a pig provides enough nutrient.

5) They consume 1.5 times more bean card than average Japanese farmers. Isoflavone found in soy bean products is recognized as preventive food for heart diseases, breast cancer, prostate cancer and such in the United States, so the effect of consuming soy beans is big.

6) Villagers eat 3 times as many green and yellow vegetables and fruit than average Japanese farmers. It is partly due to a mild climate, and fresh vegetables grow all year around.

7) As it is surrounded by the sea, fish and seaweed are always served on the table. Sermon, mackerel, tuna fish are high in Omega 3 fatty acid, and they tend to lower the risk of people suffering from heart disease, breast cancer and such.

8) The elderly people who eat traditional Okinawan food are healthy, but many young Okinawans prefer American fast food today. Due to this fact, the rate of obesity, heart disease, and those who die young are higher than those in Japan. Similarly, there has been a report that former Okinawans who immigrated to Brazil stopped eating traditional Okinawan food and switched to meat centered life. Their life span shortened an average of 17 years.

The above research proves how important it is for health to eat right.

## American style meal vs. Japanese style meal
## Hamburger vs. Japanese set meal

A typical Japanese breakfast which includes white rice, miso soup with seaweed and scallion, salmon fillet, boiled spinach season with soy sauce with a total of 452 Kcal is used as an example. On the other hand, a typical American breakfast includes 1 cup of cereal, 1 cup of milk, 1 cup of coffee or orange juice. Unlike Japan, there are many kinds of cereals. Japanese breakfast is well balanced, and the difference between Japanese and American dinner becomes remarkable. The basis of Japanese meal is rice, and there is a main dish with either fish or meat, a side dish with boiled and seasoned food or vinegar food, salad or vegetables seasoned with soy sauce.

Japanese breakfast offers many varieties of dishes. American dinner varies due to its various cultural and ethnic backgrounds, but a typical dinner consists of salad, and meat as a main dish, vegetables, the most popular one being broccolis, and mashed potatoes with pasta or bread. There are many Americans who dislike vegetables, and an amount for each dish is about twice as much as what you eat in Japan. Due to the influence of currently popular Atkins Diet, some do not eat carbohydrates including bread and pasta. This diet is biased toward animal protein as they mainly consume meat.

**Not well balanced American meal**
**Too much meat and not enough vegetables**

I dealt with hospital and institution food, and now I like to review what had been served. Basically, it was centered on meat, and especially chicken and turkey were used for meals for patients or elderly people. M hospital where I had worked was well known for its ingenuity as hospital meals, and the following is one example.

Breakfast: 4 oz of orange juice, 1 banana, 1 boiled egg, hashed brown potatoes, a slice of ham, a small box of cereal with 8 oz of milk, and coffee or tea
Lunch: cranberry juice, a bowl of corn chowder, tuna salad sandwich, ice cream and coffee or tea with 4 oz of milk
Dinner: 1 cup of mushroom soup, green salad with a cup of Italian dressing, 6 oz of baked hunter chicken (baked with skin on), ½ cup of steamed spinach, 1 cup of mashed potatoes, 1 apple, 1 roll, 1 oz of margarine, 1 cup of coffee or tea, 4oz of milk. This is an ordinary meal with approximately 2000 Kcal.

I have never worked in Japanese hospitals, so I am not able to compare hospital meals in both countries. However, even if you compare with home cooked meals; one thing is obvious that vegetables are lacking in American hospital meals. There are nutritionists in hospitals who supervise meals and count calories; and yet, I thought they lacked green and yellow vegetables and fibrous vegetables. There were lettuce, cucumber and raw carrots in tuna salad, but it was not like eating vegetables. Rather, they were simply added to tuna to make a sandwich. Green salad served for dinner contained lettuce and cucumber. Even though it was cupful, the amount is much smaller when compared to boiled vegetables. Mashed potatoes are carbohydrates rather than vegetables. The only vegetable served was ½ cup of spinach. This is only an example, but generally speaking, the amounts of green and yellow vegetables or fibrous vegetables Americans eat are small.

I asked another dietitian, and she said, "If we add vegetables, patients tend not to eat them. That's why, we think of a menu that patients are likely to eat. Although their calorie intake as well as salt and water intake is restricted, heart disease or dialysis When we include ingredient that patients do not eat, they end up not getting enough calories, so we are very careful." The menu was centered around meat including beef, chicken, turkey, and varieties of potato dishes such as fried potatoes and mashed potatoes.

## Quality over Quantity—Japanese meals

The following is an example of Japanese meals. This is also an ordinary standard meal with 2000K cal.

Breakfast: toast with jam, 1 boiled egg, boiled broccoli with 100 g of mayonnaise, 5 strawberries, 100 g of yogurt
Lunch: a bowl of rice (160 g), ginger-flavored slices of grilled pork (70 g), tomato and cabbage salad, miso soup with wakame (soft seaweed)
Dinner: a bowl of rice (160 g), broiled salmon (1 slice), hijiki (seaweed) boiled and seasoned with cooked carrots and deep-fried bean curd, spinach seasoned with soy sauce, miso soup with tofu and daikon(Japanese radish)

When compared with American meals, the consumption of dairy products, milk for instance, is a little. However, there are many varieties of vegetable dishes, and meat and fish are alternately served while different kinds of seaweed are included in the menu. Even though Americans need to take supplements for consuming Omega 3 fatty acid, Japanese meals provide it through the food. Compared to American meals, it takes longer to prepare for Japanese meals. Nevertheless, Japanese meals have the characteristics of being well balanced with each dish is laid out appetizingly and aesthetically. There are a number of different dishes, but the amount of each main dish is smaller than American dishes. When nutritional values are compared, the differences become apparent.

Living overseas is very stressful; because of that, we should include Japanese meals in our lives and maintain health. Health is based upon what you eat, and this concept is universal throughout the world.

## Losing Weight by eating brown rice

Non refined grain: A guide line for eating which was revised on January 2005 pointed out the importance of consuming non refined grain. *American Journal of Public Health*, March 2006 issue, reported the following. Research on 308,000 women between the ages 55 to 69 was conducted in the state of Iowa. The comparison was made between one group of women who had eaten more than a bowl of brown rice and the other who had not. Those who had eaten reduced death rate by 15% for vascular heart diseases. Grain contains anticancer substances and stabilizes blood sugar levels. In supermarkets, there has been an increase of products of which labels indicate that they are made of whole wheat and whole barley. It is especially noticeable in cereal and bread, and even some sushi is made with brown rice. Non refined grain is more fibrous and maintains a healthy stomach. Furthermore, the digestive and absorbing process of non refined grain takes longer than refined rice or wheat, so you feel full longer, and a desire to eat often is not likely to occur. After I changed to brown rice, I felt full with eating a half amount of white rice. When I could not reduce my weight, I changed to brown rice. After that, my bowels were active, and there was a time that I lost 7 lb (3 kg) per week. Non refined grain is an ace in the hole for me as a dieter; it is beneficial to eat it when you cannot lose weight no matter what you do.

# CHAPTER 3

# Eat Ame-Japa Meal against being fat with a Big Belly

## Escape from Metabolic Syndrome

### Pay special attention if your stomach protrudes

I was fat around the stomach which was caused by internal organ fat, and this condition is known as a metabolic syndrome. There are different patterns of fatness; some are apple shaped top fat and others are pear shaped bottom fat around which fat is centered a hip or stomach. In reality, it is not that simple. Some are simply portly or others have accumulated fat around shoulders and stomachs. However, there is a marked tendency of heavy people having internal organ fat around a stomach. The criterion for deciding fatness is that you measure the most protruding part of your stomach, and if that is within 90cm, there is no problem. If it is over 90cm, the possibility of your having internal organ fat is real. The Japanese criterion is a bit loose since it is 85cm as opposed to 90cm in the United States. The criterion is different in each country, and yet a fat stomach tends to bring about many life-style related diseases. So, it is a common desire in every country to resolve this issue quickly. Compared to fat attached to a hip or a thigh, those attached to a stomach is directly related to internal organ fat, so it is most dangerous. The measurement around my stomach was more was 1m, which indicated that I was suffering from internal organ fat, and I was half into a metabolic syndrome.

The criteria of having a metabolic syndrome is as follows: over 150 natural fat, under 40 mg/dl of HDL which is good cholesterol, over 130 mmHg blood pressure during deflated period, over 85 mmHg blood pressure during expanded period, over 150 mg/dl triglyceride, over 110 mg/dl blood sugar when hungry. If you meet two criteria, you are diagnosed as suffering from a metabolic syndrome.

Types who might fall into a metabolic syndrome are as follows: 1) you eat until you are full, 2) you never miss snacks between meals 3) it is unthinkable to cook without sugar, so you always cook with sugar, 4) you do not like green vegetables or you do not eat vegetables, 5) you love ice cream, 6) you always have nighttime snack or have a drink at night.

All but 4) was applicable to me. Regardless of your age, if the protruding part of your stomach is over 90 cm, you had better self check the six items shown above. If applicable, it is better to start from there.

## Meals to remove the fat around your stomach

The fat around a stomach tends to be a cause of a metabolic syndrome. The risk factor is high, but it is said to be easier to remove it then the fat around a thigh or a hip. I tried to remove fat around my stomach both from an eating habit and exercises.

Considering the following five things, I made a menu.

1) Try to eat a lot of high fiber vegetables
2) Reduce lipids
3) Reduce the amount of carbohydrates, mainly bread or rice, from dinner
4) Eat dinner early
5) Eat sesame seeds and such which contain a lot of magnesium

As vegetables are high fiber and calories are low, it naturally restricts the intake of calories. As I said in the section of brown rice, food fibers cause the process of digestion and absorption slow within a body, and the feeling of fullness lasts longer while it prevents overeating. Moreover, as you need to chew well when eating high fiber food, the sign of feeling full is communicated to brains and restrains appetite.

It is important to avoid cooking with oil; instead you should steam, boil, roast and sear food. Needless to say, the more oil you intake, the more oil tends to adhere around internal organs.

When there is only a short time after eating dinner, the food is not resolved and is stored as fat within a body. As often said, it is best not to sleep at least 4 hours after having dinner. You should not eat snack or have a drink 3 to 4 hours before your bed time. By eating dinner early, it avoids accumulation of fat. I tend to overeat dinner, but if you reduce eating a bowl of rice (165g-200 g), internal organ fat may be effectively reduced.

The relationship of occurrence between eating habits and a metabolic syndrome was researched by Northwestern University for 15 years. It found out that those who take a lot of magnesium tend not to suffer from a metabolic syndrome by 30% when compared with those who take a little amount of magnesium. Magnesium tends to prevent the collection of internal organ fat. The minimum amount of magnesium you should consume per day is 300mg, and sesame, seaweed, beans, and green and yellow vegetables contain a lot of magnesium. It is easy to include magnesium in your meal if you are a little bit creative. You might like to eat a sesame bagel and bread, or you might sprinkle furikake* over rice,

(Furikake*—a tastily seasoned dried food for sprinkling over rice)

It is necessary to exercise in order to remove internal organ fat. To put it another way, you can remove internal organ fat by exercising. At first, you practice aerobic exercise for 30 to 60 minutes. I recommend that you walk a little fast. What is important is that you should find some exercise that you enjoy and stick to it. After continuing a month, internal organ fat starts to burn off and doing exercise becomes easier. Three months after the start of exercise, you are no longer satisfied by just walking. It changes to jogging or you might run, and your body is ready to move up to the next level. Now, you use a suitable exercise machine two or three times a week and strengthen exercise. After half a year or so later, it is likely that your internal organ fat changes to muscle.

## Importance of Serving Meals on Dishes

It is important to serve meals correctly. I used to put food on a big plate, but as I began dieting, I changed using a big plate to a smaller plate. I serve one portion on a small plate; if I serve on a big plate, I simply overeat. Furthermore, if food is placed in front of me, I end up eating it. At first, I rigorously placed rice, a fish fillet, chicken bread on a scale and weighed them. However, my trained eyes soon recognized that a bowl of rice for women contains about 150 g of rice, and a fish fillet equal to the palm of my hand is about 3 oz.

## American Style Japanese Traditional Food for Diet

It is being noticed in the United States that Japanese traditional food, rice, fish and soy bean products lower cholesterol and reduces the risks of heart diseases. Dr. Craig Willcox, who had researched Okinawan food, says that Okinawan food can be acquired in the United States. It is not likely to get the same ingredient as in Japan, but you can obtain the same type or constituent parts of food. Even though it is very close to Japanese style food, we utilize the food in Europe especially that of Mediterranean coastal area because of olive oil and the United States, that would be an ideal American style food. To prevent the number one killer of Americans, heart diseases, to increase immunity against cancer, and to live longer, we can start by eating the following 10 longevity foods which were introduced in the nationwide newspaper, USA Today: non refined grain, fish, tea (green or black), nuts, tomato, olive oil, grapes (red), spinach, garlic, and blueberry. They are healthy food and are suitable for diet.

Fish: *British Medical Journal* has reported that two years have been spent by conducting a follow-up survey of two thousand people who had experienced a heart attack. What they found out was that those who ate fish twice a week reduced the sudden death by 23%.

According to *Journal of the American Medical Association* (January 1998 issue), research was conducted on two million 40 to 84 year old men. It found out that the risk of death caused by the sudden death by a heart attack was reduced by 52%. It is said that Omega-3 fatty acid contained in fish prevents the congealment of blood and circulate blood smoothly.

Tea (green or black tea): The effect of antioxidation is the same whether it is green or black tea. When you drink a cup of tea, it is said that the risk of heart diseases is reduced by half. Similarly, an anti-oxidant, flavanoid, is said to reduce the oxidation of cholesterol. Especially EGCG (Epigallocatechin-3-gallate) contained in green tea restrains enzyme needed to propagate cancer, and it activates cells.

Nuts: Clinical research conducted by Harvard University reported that a group that ate more than 5 ounces per week reduced the death rate by heart attack by 40%, compared to a group that did not eat any nuts. Nut's fat is unsaturated fatty acid and is Omega 3 fatty acid.

Tomato: Carotenoid and licopen contained in tomatoes are antioxidizers and reduce heart diseases by half as well as reducing a cancer risk. It was reported on *Journal of the national Cancer Institute* by Harvard University research team.

Olive oil: It was reported that due to anti-oxidation contained in olive oil, the death rate of heart attack patients were reduced by half. It became a big hit in the United States as the Mediterranean food in 2004.

Grapes (red): The anti-oxidizing power of red grape juice is more than 4 times of orange juice and tomato juice. It is also well known to lower the risk of having a heart attack. Risks related to coronary diseases are lowered, and it controls the oxidation of cholesterol.

Spinach: It is known for anti-oxidizing power. As it contains folic acid, it is effective against cancer, heart diseases, and mental diseases.

Garlic: It is known for anti-oxidizing power, and it is effective against cancer, heart diseases, and illness caused by aging. In order to reduce cancer risk, it is necessary to eat over 18g of garlic.

Blueberry: It contains antioxidant, and it is recognized for the prevention of aging including a memory decline and such. It is also found out that the growths of enzymes that speed up the division of cancer cells are restrained.

# CHAPTER 4

# Basic Meal Menu
# for flattening Stomach

### Japanese meal menu with American Ingredient

Remembering what was said in Chapter 2, let us carry on. I found out my ways after several attempts. These are my meal plans which were most suitable to me, and I escaped from being fat. Food is a matter of preference; some like it hot and some do not. When you make your own meal plans, your diet becomes close to success.

### Traditional Japanese meal style

The traditional Japanese breakfast is as follows: steamed rice, Miso soup, grilled salmon or fish, Daikom oroshi (Grated radish), and Oshinko (pickled vegetable with rice bran). Basically, white rice, miso soup with vegetable, for example, daikon (white radish), eggplant, green beans, scallion, spinach, and Tofu(beans curds), wakame (seaweed). Main dish has protein; egg, fish, hams; Side dishes have salad, oshinko, oshitashi(boiled vegetable), or Daikon oroshi(Grated radish) and fruit. Total calories are about 300kcal.

### Basic Japanese Healthy meals

If you master these basic Japanese meals, you can arrange variety of meal by yourself. Let's try it!

**Salad**
**For every body, good for the vegetarian**

**a) Su-no-mono /Seaweed Salad**

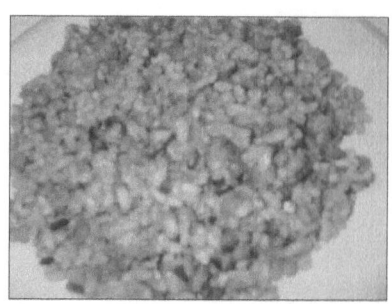

Materials: cucumber 1, Wakme (dry seaweed) 50g (1grasp), Vinegar 3 TBS, Sugar 1TBS, Soy sauce 1 TS, Salt 1/2 TS

How to make:

1) Wakame (Seaweed) soaked into water for 5-10minutes.
2) Cucumber cut to slice with little salt.
3) Vinegar, sugar, soy sauce mixed and make the vinegar sauce.
4) Mixed 1)wakame and 2)cucumber with 3)sauce.

**Rice**

**b) Brown Rice with red beans**
**For every body, good for the vegetarian**

Materials:
Sweet Rice 3cups, Red beans 1/2cup, kuro Gama (Black sesame)1/2TS, salt 1/8TS.

How to make:

1) Red beans soaked into water for overnight.
2) Red beans boiled until soften inside (about 1-2 hours). I use a pressure cooker to boil the red beans for 3minutes.
3) Washed rice and put on the basket. (Cut the water)
4) After boiled, you can use the soup of red beans. Add the red beans soup (the soup is not enough 3cups, you adjust the water to 3cups and add 3) of rice on the pot.
   (I use rice cooker to cook rice with red beans. The traditional way, the red beans rice cooks by steamed, but I introduced way is so easy to cook.)
5) Cook for 15-20 minutes, after finish to heat, keep the cover of pan about 5-10 minutes.
6) Serve the dish (bowl) and chip Kuro game and salt on the Red beans rice.

### c) Bamboo Shot Rice
### For regular meal

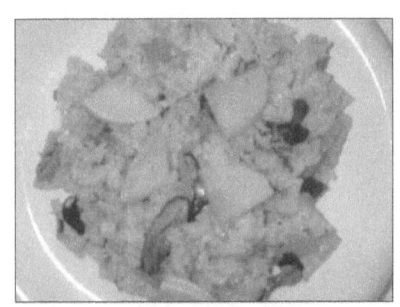

Materials:

Rice 3cups, Chicken (lean meat) 200g (1/2 lbs), Bamboo Shot 1 Carrot small 1/2,

Dry Shiitake Mushroom 2, soup 3.5 cups (Soy sauce 3TBS, Sugar 2TBS, Salt 1TS, Sake or Mirin 1 TBS, Water 3.5 cups).

How to make:

1) Chicken, Bamboo shot, Carrot wash and cut to the slice (small size).
2) Dry shiitake mushroom soaked for 10-15 minutes. After soften, cut small portion.
3) Put 1) and 2) materials on the pan, add soup 3.5cup. Cook for 3-4 minutes.
4) Move 3) to basket, use the soup for cooking the rice. Keep the materials without soup.
5) Wash the rice and put rice on the other pan with 4) soup. If the soup is not 3.5cup, adjust to the water and you can make total 3.5cups of water. (I use rice cooker in this process.)
6) Cook for 15minutes, after stop the fire, 4) materials put on the pan (rice cooker) and keep warm for 10 minutes.
7) Mix the materials with rice.
8) Serve the bowl.

*Without chicken, or use fried bean curds instead of chicken, the vegetarian use it.

### Main or side dishes

### d) Hijiki (Simmered dished)
### For every body, good for the vegetarian

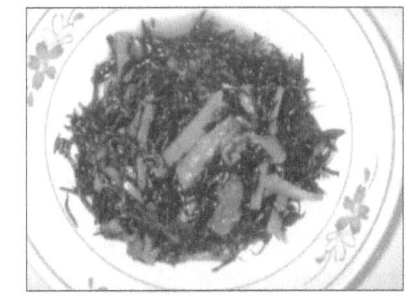

Materials:

Hijiki (seaweed) 30g, Carrot 1/2(30g), Fried bean curds(Abura age) 1 piece, Vegetable oil 1TBS, soup 1cup(water 2/3cups, sake 1TBS, Soy sauce 2TBS, Mirin 1TS, ).

How to make:

1) Dried Hijiki soak for 5 minutes and dry up.
2) Carrot and Fried bean curds cut into small strips.
3) Put vegetable oil on the pan, and heat.
4) Add 2) carrot and Fried beans curds, and fried.
5) Add soup and cook for 10 minutes.

e) **Kinhira gobo (Simmered dished)**
**For every body, good for the vegetarian**

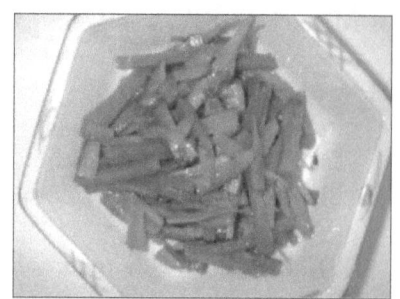

Materials:
Gobo (burdock root) 1, Carrot 1, Vegetable oil 3TBS, Soup 1cup, A {soy sauce 1/3 cup, sake 1 TBS, Mirin 1TBS (use sugar 2TBS instead of Mirin)}

How to make:

1) Gobo cut into small strips (1.5inches), and soak chopped Gobo in water.
2) Carrot cut into 1.5inches strips.
3) Heat vegetable oil on pan, add 1) gobo and 2) carrot, and stir-fried.
4) Add soup and A materials, cook for 5-7minutues.
5) Soup is gone mostly, stop the fire.

f) **Chicken Teriyaki**
**For regular meal (Not vegan)**

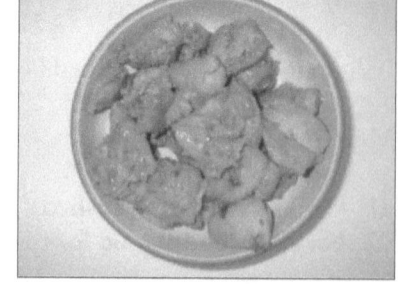

Materials:
Chicken thigh 2 pieces (3lbs-5lbs), Sauce (Soy sauce 2TBS, Mirin 2TBS), Vegetable oil 1TBS,

How to make:

1) Stab chicken by folk or knife.
2) Cut 1) chicken to small portion.
3) Heat pan and put on vegetable oil, grill 2) chicken until turning brown (both sides).
4) After brownish chicken, change to small fire and add sauce on the pan.
5) Boil down until sauce is gone.

**g) Nira Itame (Leek stir-fried)**
**For every body, good for the vegetarian**

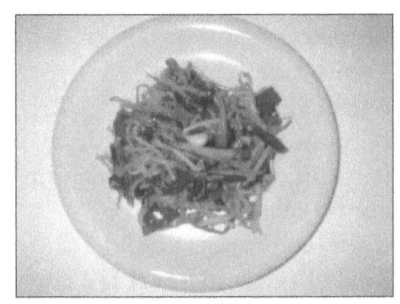

Materials:
Nira(Leek) 1bunch(1/2lbs), Moyashi
(bean sprout) 1/4 lbs(100g), garlic 1piece, sale
1/8TS, pepper 1/8TS, vegetable oil 1 TBS.

How to make:

1) Wash Nira and Miyashi. Put into the basket and off the water.
2) Cut off the root of nira (1/2inches), and cut into 2inches each.
3) Heat pan and put on vegetable oil, add crush garlic, fried.
4) Add nira and moyashi into pan, and stir-fried by high heat.
5) Add sale and pepper after cook.

# *Weekly menu
**Sunday**
**Breakfast**
**Bagel 1/2 with peanut butter**
**Egg (sunny side up) 1**
**Vegetable stir fried 1/2 cups**
**Potato 3pieces**
**Tomato 1/8**
**Coffee**
**Soy milk 1 cup**

**Lunch**
**Soba noodle 1cup**
**Tororo (Grated Yam) 1cup**
**Tare (Soy sauce and dashi soup) 1/2 cups**
**Scallion slices 1 TBS**
**Kimuchi (tsukemono) 2TBS**

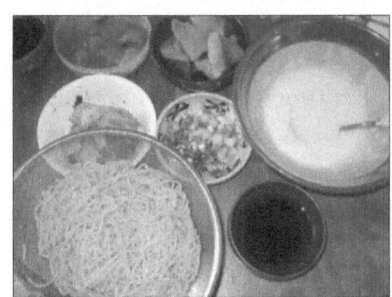

Dinner
White rice 1cup
Saba (Mackerel) grilled 1/2
Nimono, Kimpoira (basic e), chikuzennni
(daikon, shintake mushroom, fried bean
curds) each 1cup
Tofu (cole beans curds) 1/2
Tororo (Grated Yam) 1/2 cups
Seaweed salad (basic a)

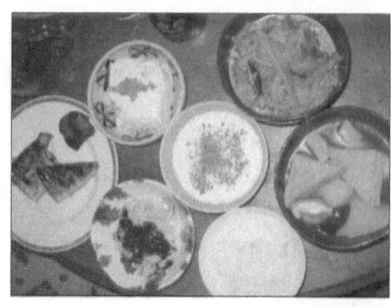

Monday
Breakfast
Toasted bread with butter 1
Yogurt 1
Soup 1cup
Apple 1
Coffee 1 cup

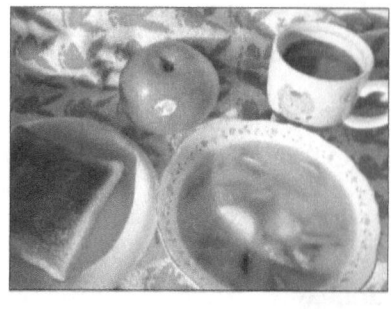

Lunch
Red Beans rice (basic b) 1cup
Saba (mackerel) grilled 1/4
Vegetable stir fried 1/2 cups
Umebashi (Pickled plum) 1

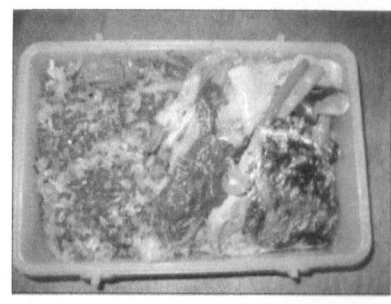

Dinner
Stir fried rice 1cup
Chicken teriyaki (basic f) 1 piece
Miso Soup (daikon wakame) 1cup
Nimono(simmered Dished) Eggplant, onion and pepper. 1cup
Seaweed salad (basic a) 1cup

Tuesday
Breakfast
Butter roll with peanut butter 1
Miso Soup (wakame, Shiitake mushroom, cabbage) 1cup
Yogurt 1
Banana 1

**Lunch**
White rice 1 cup
Chicken Teriyaki (basic f) 1 piece
Hijiki (simmered dished) (basic d) 1/2 cups
Vegetable, green beans and shiiteke mushroom nimono (simmered dished)
1/2 cups
Ginger (pickled) 2pieces

**Dinner**
Bamboo shot rice (basic c) 1 cup
Cod (1piece) steamed with carrot, celery, and sprout.
Nimono (radish, shiitake mushroom, kelp) 1cup
Soybeans simmered dished (with kelp) 1 cup

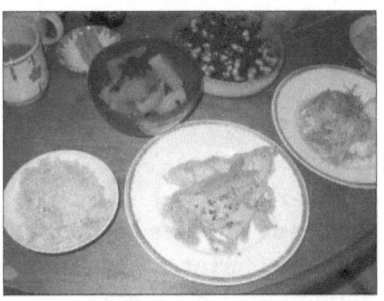

**Wednesday**
**Breakfast**
Bread 1/2
Omelet 1
Salad 1cup
Coffee 1
Orange 1
Soy milk 1 cup

**Lunch**
Bamboo Shot rice (basic c) 1cup
Cod grilled 1piece
Soybeans simmered dished 1cup
Green beans stir fried 1/2 cups

**Dinner**
Red Beans Rice (basic b) 1cup
Salmon grilled 1 piece
Nimono: carrot, radish, lutes, and fried
bean cords (simmered dished) 1cup

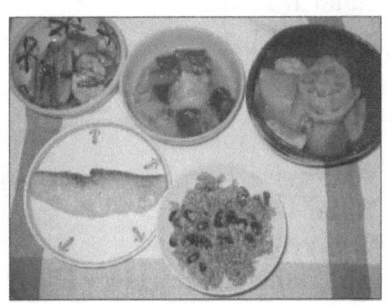

Su-no-mono(cucumber, wakame and mushroom with vinegar) 1/2 cups
Eggplant with miso taste 1/2 cups

Thursday
Breakfast
Bagel 1/2
Omelet with green 1
Salad 1/2 cups
Apple 1
Coffee 1 cup
Yogurt 1

Lunch
White rice 1cup
Soybeans simmered dished 1/2 cups
Nimono (carrot, radish, lutes, and fried bean cords) 1cup
Salmon grilled 1 piece

Dinner
Curry (A kind of stew, tasted curry included potato, carrot, onion and beef) 1cup
With white rice 1cup
Salad (lettuce, tomato, cucumber, and celery) 1cup

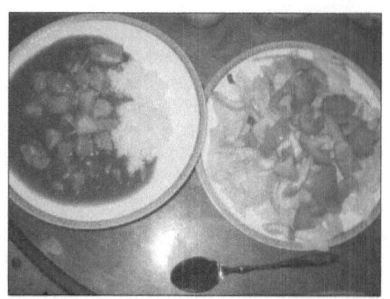

Friday
Breakfast
Toasted bread 1piece
Curry stew 1 cup
Salad 1/2 cups
Soy milk 1 cup

Lunch
White rice 1 cup
Hijiki 1/2 cups
Beef grilled 3 oz
Nira itame (basic g) (stir fried) 1/2 cups

**Dinner**
Red beans rice 1 cup
Steamed white fish with vegetable, carrot
and celery in aluminum foil
Seaweed Salad (basic a) 1 cup
Miso Soup (tofu, wakame, green pea)
1cup

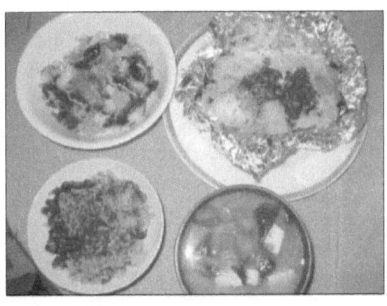

**Saturday**
**Breakfast**
Western omelets 1
Handmade bread (whole weed and nuts) 1piece
Salad ((lettuce, tomato, cucumber, onion, and celery) 1cup
Miso Soup(Seaweed, vegetable)
Kiwi 1
Soy milk 1 cup

**Lunch**
Sara udon (Stir fried Noodle with seafood
soup: shrimp, fish cakes, white fish, green
pea, onion, and carrot) 1cup
Tomato salad 1/2 cup
HIjiki (basic d) 1/2 cups

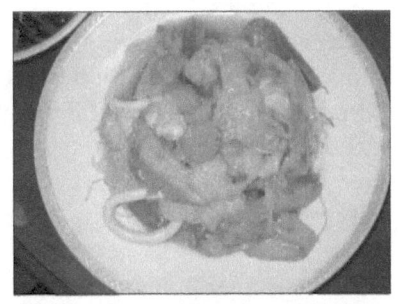

**Dinner**
Nabe (cook in the pot)
White fish (cod, red snapper,) 1 (1lbs),
Daikon (Radish) 1/2, Chinese cabbage
1/4, scallion 1bunch, Tofu 1, Shiitake
mushroom 5-6, shellfish 5-6. (You can use
for the Nabe that anything you want to
cook, some one use chicken or park instead
of fish, we do not have any rule to cook).

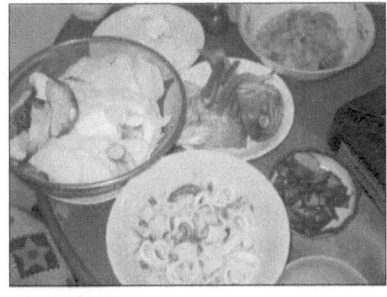

We have a lot of variety of Nabe, Yosenabe(vegetables and meat, fish boiled
with sauce), Sukiyaki(beef and vegetable in the soy sauce), Shabu shabu(boiled
thin meat and vegetables), Yudotu(boiled tofu and vegetable),

# Chapter 5

# Effect of Supplement for Diet

Having dieted myself, I learned the basics of diet: I should stop overeating, exercise and lose body fat. It is essential to eat right food, but when you see no effect, taking supplement might help your diet. It will stimulate the internal body system and help promote losing weight. Women may not realize this, but hormone tends to lose their balance as they approach the age around 50 due to menopause. Because of unbalanced hormone, it becomes harder for women to shed fat. In other words, it is not a bad idea to promote metabolism with the use of supplement. By so doing, it becomes easier for your body to shed fat.

There are supplements that you might like to take in the United States, and those especially effective for diet are listed below. Some of them are already well known in Japan. However, they are reasonably priced and have more contents compared to ones sold in Japan. They are often sold as a singular component supplement which does not contain any other substance.

## Alpha Lipoic Acid

α lipoic acid, otherwise known as thioctic acid, is a kind of supplemental enzymes and has been in use more than 30 years in the West. It is an essential component to generate energy for body metabolism, citric acid cycles, carbohydrate metabolism and such. It is also produced within a body. As it is antioxidant, it is an excellent aid to remove active oxygen which is a factor for life-style related diseases. It promotes the rate of glucose consumption which is beneficial for diet. It also works against the aging process due to the restraint of active oxygen, and it is a popular item in the United States. It is recommended to take 100mg of α lipoic acid in the United States, and it is included in many supplements for the purpose of diet, beauty treatments, and health. Recently, there is a great interest as diet material to replace Ephedra.

It became very well known in Japan as a TV program televised it. Since the Ministry of Health, Labor and Welfare officially acknowledged the indication of supplement in food in 2006, α lipson became a synonym of a diet concept. The demand of α lipson in Japan is quite big, and its use spread to cosmetics. I too am using this supplement as I learned it to be effective against aging. You take one capsule a day for three months, and the cost is about $10.00 for 120 capsules in the United States. It is no hardship!

## L-Carnitine

It is a class of amino acid produced within a body, and it promotes to burn body fat. As it takes Calnichin uses glucose and free fatty acid within muscle, it takes an important role. It is an ingredient to burn up and gets rid of unnecessary fat in a body.

It has been noticed in the United States for treating heart diseases. It is especially effective for the treatment of heart diseases which ranks as the number one cause of death.

As it is also effective for the prevention of a heart attack, it might be used with prescribed medicine by a doctor. It has been reported to ease the symptom of angina pectoris, irregular pulse and such. It often improves the condition of heart patients as well as preventing a healthy heart. The development and research are to be conducted for the prevention of hyperlipemia and the problem of the vascular system. As it is difficult to consume from food alone, taking a supplement is recommended. It is said that 1000mg of L-Calnichin per day is taken in the United States, a leading country of supplements.

Since deregulation took place in November of 2003, L-Calnichin is allowed to be used as food in Japan.

## Hoodia

Hoodia has been reported by Lesley Stahl of a long running TV program "60 Minutes" in the United States. Since then, Hoodia became an enormous hit. It is a plant resembling cactus grown in Kalahari Desert in South Africa. Bushmen, the original inhabitants of the region, have been eating it when they go out hunting. Stahl actually visited the spot and tasted brown hoodia grown in the desert and covered with thorns. She had reported that it tasted like a cucumber and did not taste that bad. She also did not become hungry all day.

Many diet products using Hoodia gordonii extraction have been sold in the United States. People who used products said, "I did not feel hunger for days. It was comfortable." Others said, "When you take it before you have a meal, you are no longer interested in eating." This seems to indicate that your appetite is decreased and you lose weight. FDA has not approved its safety yet. As this suppresses appetite, I have not taken.

## GCA (coffee beans)

GCA is initials of Green Coffee Antioxidants. It is extirpated from raw coffee beans, and Americans paid attention to GCA. A large amount of chlorogenic acids contained in coffee beans and tea works to restrain the carbohydrate which had been taken in to be absorbed into the body, and it helps to maintain glucose value. Chlorogenic acids promotes anatioxidation to maintain good health. It also helps maintain the correct value of cholesterol, lower the oxidation of bad cholesterol, and maintain the health of heart which is the number one cause of death in the United States.

According to the research conducted on animals, it has found out that anti-oxidation in the body further increases when polyphenol is increased. It has been made into a product as a "Carb Crasher" and such in the United States. GCA lowers the absorption of carbohydrate taken by way of food and helps burn body fat, and it is very popular in the United States.

New products made of coffee, cocoa and green tea which contains a lot of polyphenol known for oxidation has been commercially successful. As "Specified Health Food" indicates, GCA, extracted from raw coffee beans, is highly noticed as dieting ingredients.

I love green tea, and I always drink at least 4 or 5 cups of green tea both in the morning and at night, so I do not feel like taking GCA from supplements. Even though some Americans drink coffee as if there is no tomorrow, they feel they do not take in enough polyphenol and still take supplements. Burning fat, absorbing and extracting fat, and preventing to resolve carbohydrate is the objectives of these supplements. It is necessary to select supplements depending upon your bodily constitution and the type of fatness. Ingredients to burn body fat have become popular recently.

## Multiple Vitamin and Minerals

Basically it is best to get vitamins and minerals from food, but it becomes harder to compound and resolve them after you become middle age. So, it becomes necessary to supply vitamins as supplements. As I turned to 50 years old, I began taking a multiple vitamin a day. As you become middle aged, in order to lose weight healthily, it becomes necessary to have an aid of supplements such as vitamins and minerals.

# CHAPTER 6

## Importance of Exercise. Try a few . . .

I did not mind dieting, but I did not want slacken skin as well as increased wrinkles. After dieting, you might look older as your skin might dry out. Dieting with food only may cause this condition. In order to lose weight youthfully and healthily, it is effective to combine exercise with diet.

It is recommended that you choose your favorite exercise that you can do.

### New York City offers an Affordable Gym
### Recommending municipal Recreation Center

Places where I can use a pool are fairly limited in Manhattan. Of course you can obtain anything in this country if you can pay for it, but it is impossible for me to go to gyms where I have to pay a high entrance fee. It is convenient to use public facilities. I live in Chelsea in Manhattan, and there is Chelsea Recreation Center where I live. There are a basement and 6 floors equipped with a gym, table tennis, and a 50m swimming race indoor pool. (430 West 25th Street, NYC 10001/212-255-3705) Because it is a municipal gym, the admission fee is $75 (18-55 years old), and if you are over 55 years old, it is only $10 annually. There are 15 other municipal recreation centers. Once you join in one recreation center, you can use any recreation centers. New York City is divided into 5 sections, which are Manhattan, Bronx, Brooklyn, Queens, and Staten Island. There are a total of 55 Recreation Centers, and they are as follows: 12, 8, 10, 5, and 5 in Bronx, Brooklyn, Queens, Staten Island, and Senior Center respectively. In order to become a member, you need to bring something with a picture to identify yourself, and you can become a member right there. Upon paying the admission fee, you can use a swimming pool and a gym without fee. As perhaps the city does not advertise, there are many Americans who do not know about it. Even YMCA considered reasonably priced charges the admission fee of $120 and a monthly fee of $75, so you need to pay $1020 annually. Even though there are much better facilities for yoga classes and slimming exercises in private gyms or YMCA, I choose inexpensive fees anytime. For those who do not want to spend much money, I recommend reasonable municipal centers. I myself joined at once.

### Aqua walking removes belly fat?

I began with a pool. It sounds as if I am very good at swimming, but actually, swimming is not really my strong point. Rather than swimming, I started to walk in the water. As if I was rehabilitating, I walked from one shallow end to the other shallow end of the pool. At first, it looked easy, but unlike walking on the ground, I strained at my stomach due to water pressure. Once your body gets used to it, you can jog, raise your leg high, shake an arm or run in the water.

I remembered when I took a water aerobics class. It is the exercise done in water. You wrap a belt made of Styrofoam around your body and carry a dumbbell also made of Styrofoam in your hand. Listening to hip-hop music in the background, it is enjoyable to move your body. You try an hour per week, and it is effective for the prevention of gaining weight while I enjoyed a change of pace. Then, I decided to do this by myself.

Although other people were swimming, I wrapped a Styrofoam aqua belt around the body. The aqua belt is for water exercise. I was initially embarrassed to do such exercises as riding a bicycle, scissor exercises, jumping with both legs open, and water jogging. But, this is America. Unlike Japan, you do not have to worry about what other people think of you that much. Besides, I really do not pay much attention what others think about me. I moved my body sufficiently in my own pace. However, as it is very cheap, the pool schedule was not always convenient for me.

### Schedule you weekly exercise schedule

The exercising guidance issued by the Government suggests that we exercise three times a week for 60-90 minutes, but 60 minutes is simply to maintain health. At least, you need to exercise for 90 minutes. It is important that you get used to exercise, so I decide to do every day rather than three times a week. I swam when it was available for me, and I searched for such suitable sports as yoga, pirates, jogging, and such for the days swimming was not available.

It is pretty hard to continue water exercise on my own. Once you miss one day, you tend to pamper yourself and become lazy. In New York City, especially in Manhattan, much yoga, gym and such classes for beginners are available.

## Activate metabolism by Practicing Hot Yoga

Hot yoga got into the limelight in 2006. You exercise yoga poses for 90 minutes in the room where the wind as hot as 100 degrees blows. There was a trial course that you pay only $20 for one hour course and take as many classes as you can, so I invited my friend for a trial class. A minute after I entered the room, I started to sweat. Women wearing tank tops or swim suits or men naked from waists up keep enough space for a yoga mat. The room was filled with hot air. An instructor gave a command but did not show yoga poses in details, and students were simply imitating others. I could not perform many yoga poses, and I realized that how I could not perform any poses due to the lack of exercise. Bu looking at the mirror, I truly acknowledged that how fat I have become. My hand could not touch the floor because of my belly fat, and I could not raise my body as I lacked abdominal muscle. Since my balance was way off, I wobbled as I tried to stand on one foot. There was not a single pose that I could practice. The instructor assured me, "If you continue for three months, you will lose weight." So, after finishing the trial practice, I purchased a book of tickets for which $15 is charged per session. I went to yoga practice once a week for three months. It was certainly effective, but I could not afford $15 per session. I practiced the poses I had learned at home, but it was not heated and I did not sweat. I could not expect the same effectiveness as found in class.

Since I heard that yoga was good for diet, I participated in many other yoga classes. The fee was around $15-25 for one 90 minute lesson. After practicing hot yoga, it was not quite satisfactory as I did not sweat as much. I could not perform many poses since I was had a fat belly, and I did not get expected results. If I continued longer, I might have gotten better results. But if you are doing yoga for the purpose of losing weight, it is true that you do not feel like continuing it unless you see some results within three months.

## Pilates burns belly fat

Pirates have become popular last year. It is the exercise for such artists as ballerinas and dancers who use their bodies to express art. Students use machines to correct bodies. There are different levels, and a true Pirates class cost $150 to 300 per hour. When I attended a class offered by a municipal gym, it appeared to be a slimming exercise class to train abdominal muscles. There was no machine in this class, and I used an exercise mat. As I was fat and did not have abdominal muscles, it was very difficult for me to exercise this as well. First off, I could not raise my upper part of the body. Someone had to hold my legs, and I was barely able to lift my upper body. Nevertheless, I decided to continue as it was very cheap, only $60 for 10 classes. Besides, I thought it would be better to do this rather than walking on the machine. This gives me some variations as well. Apart from the instructor, every student was fat, so I felt comfortable. The main focus of Pilates class is to use abdominal muscles, so I felt as if my belly fat was trembling all over. When one session was over after three months, I still had belly fat, but my triple layered stomach fat was reduced to a double layered stomach fat. I am still continuing Pilates once a week tirelessly, and I now can do sit-ups easily, and my belly fat has changed to stomach muscle.

## Walking is economical and best for me

What you could do without feeling a burden is walking; it is most economical. I decided to use such machines as a trade mill and a bicycle. It is easy to use the trade mill as you can set up your desired walking speed, distance and course. It can also adjust the time to cool down depending on heartbeat. I adjusted the first five minutes to walking speed, and, I switched to fast walking after I felt ready. After 25 minutes, I switched to the cool down mode. I walk until I slightly sweat which is about 30 minutes. If you listen to music while doing it, time goes so quickly. Since it is a municipal gym, it is rather crowded, and some machines are not available. As a riding a bicycle machine is usually available, I just make do with it.

Since the municipal recreation center is very crowded, I joined the sports gym which belongs to my apartment building. An annual fee is $165, and the use of the gym is limited to the residents only, so it is not as crowded as the municipal center. The trade mills and bicycles in the gym are equipped with televisions, and I can exercise while watching TV as long as I bring an earphone. It is open from 6 a.m. until 11 p.m., and it became necessity for me. Here I exercise in the evening after dinner.

As there is a green park along the Hudson River, I either go for a walk or jog up to Hudson River Park when the weather is good. Since there are so many cars in Manhattan, it is rare to find a place that you can walk leisurely. Nevertheless, when you look for it, you can find a number of playgrounds or small parks. When I have time, I try to go outside and walk even for 30 minutes. Walking is most suitable exercise for me.

A greenway in New York City totals 350 miles and is expanding every year. The greenway is a trail, which is similar to a promenade in Japan, and it includes randomly located thirteen parks, two gardens, an aquarium and an art museum. You might say it is a road where you can exercise. It extends from Battery Park downtown Manhattan to 125th Street uptown Manhattan. Along the Hudson River, there is a greenway where a biker, skater, runner, and walker can use. Some areas are still under construction, and along with pleasant breeze skimming along many piers, it is nice to go for a walk on a day off. On the way, there is a bicycle rental center or a pier where you can paddle a canoe for free, and all the family members can enjoy. Besides Manhattan, greenways are established in Brooklyn and Queens as well, roughly 5 miles of roads are expanded. There are about 10 greenways including Coney Island, well known by Japanese for hotdog eating competition, Ocean side, and Alley Pond.

Inviting a few friends, you talk a walk for a couple of hours through the greenway. It is a pleasurable way to continue exercise.

# EPILOGUE

## After losing weight, there are many benefits

As I lost 55 lb. (25 kg), many things that I had not anticipated before going on a diet occurred. Pants which were so tight with my own flesh and fat became too large. I was not able to wear pants unless the elastic was sewn around waist, but now I could not wear pants without supported by a belt. My own clothes became so big, and they did not fit me anymore. I knew it was uneconomical, but I bought new clothes. Unlike before, it is fun to choose clothing. I only went to big size cloth stores; I now can choose clothes without constraint now. When I bought summer clothes, the size was 14 in 2006. It became the size 12, 10 and 8 in the fall of 2006, spring of 2007 and the summer of 2007 respectively. Even though extra large clothes are easily found in the United States where so many people are fat, there are more to choose from for regular clothes sizes, and sales associates treat you better. People commented me that I look more beautiful after losing weight, but the truth is what I wear is making a difference. I used to wear clothes that cover over my fat belly, but now I wear something more fashionable.

What has changed most after losing weight is the movement of my body. It was hard to climb up 150 subway steps when I was fat, but now I can do easily without stopping. The escalator during the morning rush hour is crowded with people, but the stairway is almost empty. Disregarding a long wait for the escalator, I run up the stairway without panting, and this gives me a little sense of superiority. A year ago, I was definitely waiting for the escalator for a long time. I used to find a seat quickly as I got on the subway, but now I no longer am concerned if I find a seat or not. Since losing weight, I do not tire easily. My belly now is flat, and no one takes me as a pregnant woman or no one offers me a seat in the subway.

Fat around my stomach prevented me to do satisfying stretching, but now I can do it easily. It was dreadful that I was carrying extra 55 lb every day. I have a full realization of being light.

After a successful diet, I realized that my sense of taste has changed. I now remove all the fat from the meat and eat mainly less fatty meat such as breast of chicken or filet. Instead of meat, I now eat whitefish and do not eat sweet food at all. I boil food with soup stock with dried kelp and soy sauce, and the flavor is simple. I use vinegar and a little bit of olive oil for vegetable salad. At first, I did not think I could eat it as it was so tasteless. Actually, I started to notice the tasty flavor of ingredients. I did not think I was cooking until I added sugar before, but now I realized the sweetness coming from daikon and carrots. Having chewed thoroughly and slowly, I felt food without adding sugar was natural and tasty. I used to tell myself that I was very busy and frequently used instant soup base and instant food.

Food is the basis for diet, and I checked my cooking closely. After going back to basics, I began cooking with Japanese traditional cooking method. Then my tongue that had lost the original taste buds was revived. It takes longer, but making miso soup with dried kelp base is very tasty. Vegetables flavored with shiitake mushrooms are not bad. We live in the world of high speed, and everything that was done speedily and quickly was considered preferable, but food is exception. As my tongue recovered the taste I had forgotten, I noticed a small amount of sugar if added while cooking and did not like it. My tongue no longer accepts food cooked with white sugar. I became sensitive to taste, and such processed food as sausage and ham are no longer my favorite. I taste chemical seasoning on my tongue, and I smell chlorine in water. I no longer want to eat meat so much. Vegetables are natural and tasty. I used to vow never to become a vegetarian as they eat only vegetables. There are so many wonderful things to eat besides vegetables. After losing weight, however, my tongue craves food close to vegetarian dishes. I now believe that the tongue is honest because a tongue wants to eat what a body needs. So, now the way I eat is simply following my tongue which has become honest.

# SUMMARY

**Seven Steps toward Successful Dieting—What you should not forget while on a Diet**

1. Change your meals and exercise. Do not be deceived by fake diets.
2. Do not give up your diet as it is important to continue. Find out what your goal is.
3. Do not expect the quick result. Expect to take the same amount of time to lose as you gained your weight.
4. When you practice, you will lose weight. If you do not practice, you will not lose weight.
5. Go back to the basics of traditional Japanese cooking, and eat well balanced meals with well balanced amounts and well balanced eating orders.
6. Do not lose weight sickly but healthily.
7. Learn how to cope with rebounds.

Before starting on a diet, I was only thinking how to lose weight. I tried this way and that. When I think about the reason why I was not successful now, the reason is very small. Do not give up as it is essential to continue. You repeat eating right meals and keep doing exercises. In order to continue, you must decide your own goal. A clue to my successful diet was that I did not want to be taken as a pregnant woman, and I was fearful of becoming ill due to a weight problem.

It is not wise to become very impatient to get results. Fasting on your own, eating only one item, pineapple for example, stop eating carbohydrates completely, or reducing the amount of food intake extremely are not healthy, and I do not recommend it. After staying on a complete diet, I felt my skin very died-up and could not put make up on well. As my face was very pale, I knew it was not a good diet. If my face began to turn pink and I can put make up on smoothly, I did not have any problem. So, I decided to manage myself better.

As you reduce your food intake extremely, the source of energy is reduced as well. Your will probably lose weight, but as your body mechanism tries to work with the limited energy, your weight will eventually end up going back to what it was. Furthermore, as I myself had experienced, by the loss of extreme food intake, you have the reaction to eat; you simply cannot stop eating. When reaction hit me, the amount of food I ate was three times as much. So, there were a few times that I gain more weight than before I started dieting. Reviewing what you eat and reducing extra calories is important so that your weight goes back to normal, but it is never a good idea to do things extremely. As it took some time to gain weight, you need to spend the same amount of time to lose weight. Unless you are sick, you do not lose weight suddenly, and you can hurry your result. If you lose 5-10 lb. (2.5 kg) per month, you are dieting successfully. There were a few times that I could not lose weight. The result of diet varies according to people. You should not compare or compete with others, but you should believe in your losing weight. Eat traditional Japanese food and eat regularly.

There was a time that I started to lose weight again after one week or there was a time that nothing changed for one month. And yet, I started losing weight again after many trails and error. I checked the amount of food intake, changed exercises, and ate meals earlier. I calmly set my objectives for every three months without trying too hard. When you practice dieting, you will lose weight. If you do not diet, you will not lose. This simple principle is the basis of dieting, and it is important to lose healthily so that your condition is good, and you feel like ready and willing.

Unless you burn up calories you have eaten, it will be stored in your body. That is what I learned from my dietetics. My professor said that dietetics was chemistry, but I say dietetics is the chemistry of eating. In a word, you eat many kinds of correct amounts of balanced meals and eat them in the order of good balance. It is not difficult, and you simply go back to the basics of traditional Japanese meal. Staple diet is rice, and you eat with miso soup. As side dishes, you may not eat a huge amount, but you eat at least 3 kinds of vegetables, meat and soy beans. If you keep this principle, you may like to arrange Japanese food as you like. The outstanding features of Japanese food are that you can add noodles, bread and such into different kinds of menus.

Another important thing is that the amount of meal you are going to eat would be roughly half of regular American meals. Before your stomach or intestines get used to large American meal portions, you should maintain to be satisfied with Japanese meal portions. It was very difficult for me to return to Japanese meal size as I was very used to eat American meal portions.

Once you get the hang of dieting, even if you overeat, you can adjust it with smaller meals and exercises. It is not necessary to take a dim view of overeating. If you overeat, you control it by eating less next day. In case you overeat dinner, you should exercise. If I overate dinner, I fast walked around my apartment building. By just walking 30 minutes, you can resolve the problem of overeating dinner. When you master these methods of fixing overeating, you are in good hand. I no longer have an urge to eat like mad or belief that I cannot stop eating. I never felt like starving by dieting. I lost my weight slowly and gradually, and I am maintaining my weight at 120 lb (55 g)

# POSTSCRIPT

The American style Japanese meal is the conclusion I have approached after several attempts to find out what would be an effective diet. It has worked for me, but I am not certain if it works for everyone. That is to say each body system is different, and the inclination to eat a certain type of food and eating habits are different. Because of this, I cannot say my method is 100% perfect, but I have lost 20 kg by including some Japanese food into American diet. It is not drastically changing your way of eating, but you add one or two items, and you will gradually correct mistakes. This book is only a hint, and you should cook your own Japanese meals with your own creativity and device.

It is my at most pleasure if my experience is helpful for those who want to study in the U.S.A., work as an expatriate, come for private purposes, or those who have lived and become used to American food, or those who have been eating American food and have gained a lot of weight, and also Americans who want to lose weight but are not able to.

www.ingramcontent.com/pod-product-compliance
Lightning Source LLC
Chambersburg PA
CBHW021253280526
45784CB00005B/2353